THE PROCRASTINATOR'S SURVIVAL GUIDE

A Common Sense, Step-By-Step Handbook
To Prepare For and Survive Any Emergency

By BOB MAYER

This publication has been carefully researched, and is based on the author's training and experiences as well as the best available information as of the publication date. It is the advice and opinion of the author. It is intended to provide helpful and useful material on the subjects covered. The author and publisher are not engaged in rendering medical services and highly recommend a doctor be consulted on all matters that require medical attention, diagnosis or treatment. The author and publisher specifically disclaim all responsibility for any liability, loss or risk, personal or otherwise, that is incurred as a consequence, directly or indirectly, of the use and application of any of the contents of this book. Neither the publisher or author accept responsibility for any loss, injury, or damage caused as a result of techniques presented in this book; nor for any prosecutions or proceeding instigated against any person or organization resulting from use of these techniques. The reader must use their own good judgment in using the information presented. This book is sold without any warranties or guaranties of any kind, and the author and publisher disclaim any responsibility or liability for personal injury, property damage, or any other loss or damage, however caused, relating to the information in this book.

eISBN: 9781621253273
Print ISBN: 9781621253266

Task One
**_Mild: Get two cases of bottled water for each
person in your household._**

Store in a dry, shaded place.

Table of Contents

Forward by Bob's Wife
A Procrastinator and Believer in Making Luck Backwards

INTRODUCTION

PREPARATION

31   Do Your Area Study

83   Prepare the Five Key Elements for Survival

124   The Places For Which To Plan

SURVIVAL

Stockpile, Scavenge, Sustain

In Conclusion

Appendixes

Forward by Bob's Wife: A Procrastinator and Believer in Making Luck Backwards

Deb:

If you're like me, you don't buy books about surviving things. Why? Probably because you think that you won't survive them anyway, so why bother? We can call it procrastination but sometimes it's easier to think of it as something which we'd rather not think about at all.

My husband, Bob, is a person who does think about 'what's the worst that could happen' and thus frees me up to forget about that. I've always seen it as another quirky part of the man whom I've loved since I first saw his bookshelf because we had almost all of the same books.

He had the same tattered paperbacks of Asimov, Bradbury and Heinlein and on and on telling me that he, too, had spent his teenage years in worlds not this one but maybe a future this one.

He had more fantasy than I, and I had more true crime than he, but otherwise we had a matching set of bookshelves. He had a lovely special edition of Watership Down and I had a complete set of the Encyclopedia of Crime which I still consider my best buy from a library sale.

I did have an interest in 'what's the worst thing that could happen' but mine focused on the past and his is directed toward a future which oddly enough only a survivalist is optimistic enough to imagine. If you worry about how to snare a rabbit after the zombie apocalypse-- you are a glass half full person. And that means you don't need this book because you've already got a few.

But, if you're like me and rather convinced that the first person infected with zombiasm will be your orthopedic surgeon during your rotator cuff surgery and they'll just lean over and take a real chunk of you in lieu of payment, and thus end future travails, you're the odd combination of glass half empty, yet believe you'll be lucky.

The problem is that I'm not lucky and I write this because we procrastinators tend to put things off not because we're lazy or inept: rather our need for perfection prefers to wait for the proper mood. If you're still reading this then you know what I mean. There does come the perfect mood to write the paper in one sitting, to rearrange the closet, to make the photo albums and brush the dogs. People like Bob don't wait for that mood and do a bit everyday so he's always caught up on the minutiae of life. I find it unbearably unfair that he and all the people like him think this is normal because it is. It's such a common sense approach to living that my procrastination must reject it because my uncommon sense works for me. If it didn't then I wouldn't put off that which can be done today for no reason other than it makes common sense in favor of doing it when it makes uncommon sense to me.

But, there is an issue with uncommon sense in that it's a bit of magical thinking and sees luck as a real thing. Or as I sometimes call it, the magical power of negative thinking.

My meandering point here is that I didn't worry about the zombie apocalypse because I wouldn't survive the first day of it and that gave me peace for a long time. Another way of thinking of that is that I never had to be in the mood to think of survival, so I could procrastinate to my heart's content until the day that Bob burst my magical thinking by mentioning that the lucky people won't survive the first day of whatever 'worst he could imagine'.

Well, that's not good at all because he's lucky and I'm not. We procrastinators aren't stupid or lazy: we just need the mood for perfection and that day I was in the mood to hear that if I applied his theory to my magical thinking about luck and survival then the zombie eats Bob on the first day. I'll be in the bathroom and survive and crawl out the window and for the first time my mood will perfectly match the reality of the situation at hand: I will want to survive and have no clue how. Because as my walking encyclopedia of survival husband mentions from time to time, nothing makes you want to survive as much as the moment you're trapped in that bathroom and survival becomes an option.

Because that is the procrastinator's dilemma in that we'll never prepare till the mood strikes us to prepare perfectly. And that mood will, of course, never strike us till the zombies are clawing at the bathroom door. So, for everyone who ignores the improbable while also occasionally falling into the perfect mood to clean out every closet and the basement and attic all in one day because it's so easy and fun to do it now? I offer you this book and remind you that by reading it we can be assured that we'll never need it. Because that would be lucky. You know, to buy it and read it and be prepared and actually need it, too? Yeah, we're not that lucky.

In other words, we who care the least can save the world from zombies by preparing for the 'worst that we can imagine'. We who can move mountains when the mood strikes us can stop the mountains from moving by forcing ourselves to imagine that they will and prepare how to deal. Because what terrible thing will ever happen once all of us who put things off till the perfect time all know how to catch a rabbit in a snare?

Read this book and save the planet. We owe it to all the people who make lists and clean out their fridges cause it's clean-out-the-fridge day. We have the power to save them by reading this book because there will never be a day where we're in the mood to read it.

Procrastinators Unite. PU, a rather perfect term for us!

The lack of luck survey:
If you check more than three of the following items you lack luck but control that by controlling bad luck.

1. A tornado destroyed your wedding venue the day before the ceremony. (yeah, that's happened)
2. You've never experienced a toothache, fever, heart palpations or a limping dog except on Friday after five pm. (always)
3. You keep a nice tote umbrella in the car which is removed by the serviceman working on your car seat and you don't discover that until the day you get your first spray tan. (check)
4. You've never called a plumber except on a weekend when you have houseguests.
5. When you do call a plumber or any type of service person they say—"I've never seen this before."
6. You buy a new car and don't buy the wheel and tire insurance but do buy the protective coating and drive it home and have a wreck which explodes the tire and shreds the rim but there isn't a scratch on the car. (totally happened)
7. You've never once had a Kleenex when you needed one but always dig through a ton of nice Kleenex when you can't find your car keys.
8. If there is an ice storm in your area, it will be on the morning after the day you did the prep for a colonoscopy.

INTRODUCTION

Task One-again.
Mild: Did you get the two cases of water bottles
for each person in your household?

If you did, you've just taken the most important step in preparation for an emergency or natural disaster: an adequate supply of water for at least six days for each person.

If you didn't, you're still procrastinating, but you get points for continuing to read! So good news-bad news. Now get that water!

Each time you see the Special Forces patch in this book, it indicates a task you should do to prepare. These items are numbered and in a combined checklist at the end so you can keep track of how you're doing.

This book is designed for you. The person who has concerns about whether you are adequately prepared for emergencies and disasters but hasn't been able to focus on it, or when you do, quickly get overwhelmed by the information available. It is written to help you prepare for and deal with a wide array of possible situations in a common-sense, step by step manner.

We are constantly being bombarded with images of people caught in both natural and unnatural emergencies and disasters. They appear on our television screen and we watch the devastation, confusion and chaos with a combination of relief and fear. Relief because it's not us and fear because even though we bury the emotion, telling ourselves *that won't happen to us,* we know deep down that accidents, disasters and emergencies do not discriminate and can strike anyone, anywhere, at any time. You, and someone you love, will definitely face at least one of the topics covered in this book.

The key is to be prepared and this book will show you how to do it. It gives you checklists that you can readily follow in order to be ready. It also allows you to prepare by levels, from mild to moderate to extreme. Finally, it tells you what to do in various scenarios.

There are two main parts. The first is preparation. The second is survival.

Task Two
Mild: A-Team Contact Information & Alert Flow

A-Team Member	Cell Phone Number	Work/School Address & Phone #
#1		
#2		
#3		
#4		
#5		
#6		
#7		
#8		
#9		
#10		

The out of area emergency point of contact is someone who would be unaffected by a local disaster or weather event and everyone can contact to update their status. This is in case you can't contact each other in the midst of the emergency/disaster.

We'll discuss the Immediate Rally Point and Emergency Rally Point later, but for now think of the first as a place outside, but near to your house where everyone would gather if, for example, there was a fire in the home and you had to evacuate in the middle of the night.

The Emergency Rally Point is a place further away from your house, a secure location, where your family/team would gather if caught in a large scale disaster/emergency and you needed to get together. This could be a relative's home, work place, school, whatever.

Mild: Out of Area Contact, Immediate Rally Point, Emergency Rally Point

Out of area contact location, phone #	
Immediate Rally Point location	
Emergency Rally Point location	

Mild: Emergency Information

Place	Phone	Address
Poison Control	**800-222-1222**	N/A
Work #1 for ?		
Work #2 for ?		
School #1 for ?		
School #2 for ?		
Closest police station		
Closest emergency room		
Closest fire station		
Power company/ Gas company		
Water company		
Family Doctor		
Health Insurance & Account #		
Insurance company Account #		

We're on a roll. You now have more information and are more prepared than you were when you started this book. Remember, many of us don't have phone numbers memorized. We rely on the address book of our cell phone, but in an emergency, that might not work, you might not have your cell phone and have to use someone else's, or, well, as you shall see, there are many other reasons to actually have these numbers and locations written down.

Make sure everyone has an ICE (in case of emergency) phone number on their cell phone.

Android users running 7.0 or higher can program emergency information and contact details through the emergency call screen when the device is locked.

On the iPhone go to your Health App, which looks like this:

1. Launch the Health app on your iPhone.
2. Tap the Medical ID tab.
3. Tap Edit in the upper right corner.
4. Tap Edit Medical ID.
5. Under Emergency Contacts tap Add emergency contact.
6. Select a contact from your list.
7. Select a Relationship.

You can add as much information as you like on this app in the appropriate places. Think about it. If you were found unconscious and your phone is locked, could anyone contact someone who would need to know? Would medical personnel know your blood type and allergies?

To access it, when the passcode screen comes up, you will see emergency in the bottom left of that screen. Tap that and you will get a phone dial screen; on the bottom left it will say, in red, Medical ID. Tap that and you will get all the pertinent information.

WHY YOU NEED THIS BOOK

Because we know we need to do *something*, but we're not sure what, and there's just so much other stuff to do in day-to-day living we never get around to that *something* that could save our lives and the lives of the people we love.

80% of Americans live in a county that has been hit by a weather related disaster since 2007

60% of people have not practiced or prepared for what to do in an emergency

55% of people think they can rely on the "authorities" to rescue them

53% of people do not have a three day supply of water

52% of families do not have an emergency rally point (ERP)

48% of people have no emergency supplies

44% of people have no first aid kit

42% of people do not know the phone numbers of immediate family members

In the Green Berets, the most important thing that made us elite was our planning. We not only thoroughly planned our missions, we also *prepared* for all the possible things we could imagine going wrong.

You prepare for 3 reasons:
To avoid the emergency.

To have a plan, equipment, training etc. in place in case the emergency strikes.

To give you peace of mind in day-to-day living so you don't constantly have to worry about potential emergencies because you are prepared for them. This allows you to experience a higher quality of life.

Procrastination comes from the Latin: pro= forward; crastinus=belonging to tomorrow. Which is a bit redundant, but you get the point. When we procrastinate we stay in a constant state of worry, knowing there's something that needs to be done, but hasn't been. By ticking off these tasks, your peace of mind will expand.

DEFINITIONS

There are so many variables when we consider the possible disasters, emergencies, accidents, etcetera that we could face both on a day to day basis and long term. To ensure we're on the same page, let's agree on some definitions.

Three Levels of Emergencies.
I'm going to define three types of survival situations/emergencies and will use these definitions throughout the book. They are also the order of what is most likely to happen. Our immediate goal is be prepared for a mild emergency. As we go through we can just focus on mild initially, and then come back to the higher levels; when we're done procrastinating.

Mild: We experience some discomfort from our normal routine for no more than 48 hours, but it is not life threatening. Example: Our power goes off for a day or two.

Moderate: We experience a large change from our normal routine, either natural or man-made, which is not immediately life threatening but has the potential to become so if not dealt with, and/or it continues. Example: Our power goes off for five days or more. Our car slides off the road in a remote area and you are trapped inside. A powerful hurricane is approaching. A large earthquake strikes.

Extreme: A catastrophic natural or man-made event that immediately threatens our life and the lives of all around us, and if it continues, will be a constant threat. Example: A tsunami hits our coastal town. A tornado destroys our home. Nuclear, biological and chemical accident or warfare or terrorist attack. A powerful earthquake. The collapse of civilization. A pandemic with a high transmission and kill rate, aka zombies. Assume the worst until the situation stabilizes.

Length of emergency depends on how widespread it is, how severe, and how long it takes society to recover, if at all. There are too many variables to make any definitive parameters.

Some extreme emergencies could be very short in duration. For example a severe car crash. A mild emergency that continues, might have a severe, long-term effect, such as a drought that doesn't abate. There could be a slow economic failure that will take years. A mild emergency for one person could be extreme for someone else—for example a hornet sting is painful and irritating for one person but life-threatening for someone who has an adverse reaction. That is why the Area Study which we'll do is so important.

As you will see in the Area Study, I make a split and give a Mild Level of preparation and then a Moderate/Extreme (Mod/Ex) level. Initially, focus on being prepared for Mild. Then move to Mod/Ex in the priority determined by your Area Study. Mod/Ex is when you are moving from common emergencies that we all endure (such as a power outage) to something where you will probably have to evacuate your home for an indeterminate period of time. The former will certainly happen; the latter is one that is only a possibility we hope never occurs to us.

AREA OF OPERATIONS refers to the area around you. This includes your home, work, and school. It expands or contracts depending on the circumstances.

A-TEAM refers to the people you will be with during an emergency/disaster. For many of us that naturally means our family. For others, it could be a group of people we've coordinated with beforehand (more on that shortly). In an emergency it could also be the people we're trapped with. I use this term instead of constantly referring to family/team.

IRP stands for Immediate Rally Point. This is a point outside of your home where your family can gather if they have to evacuate the house for some reason. The most likely reason for this would be if there was a fire. It needs to be a place that's easily identifiable and not far from the house and everyone can find in the dark.

It's also the place where your A-Team will rendezvous if they can't go into the house for whatever reason, but need to assemble from other locations, such as school and/or work.

A street intersection near the home works well. Or a neighbor's home.

ERP stands for Emergency Rally Point. It is where everyone will assemble if they can't get to the IRP or home. This is also where your A-Team will rendezvous if they have to evacuate the home/work/school during a moderate or extreme emergency and have to stay for at least a day or more, with the possibility of not returning to the home.

BOHS stands for Bug Out Hide Site and is only for extreme emergencies where you've left your home and don't plan on coming back. It refers to being on the move and also wherever you may stop, either temporarily or permanently, depending on the extent of the emergency and threats.

GnG stands for Grab-n-Go bag.

ORGANIZATION OF THE BOOK

The overall flow is from Preparation to actual Survival.

In Preparation, the flow is from the Area Study through more specific information about the five elements of survival to the places for which to plan, the places to plan for, and then Grab-n-Go bags which transitions us into actual Survival information.

Under Survival we cover the first five things to do in an emergency to the key phrase to keep in mind in an emergency, SURVIVAL, to first aid, water and food procurement, shelter and fire, and then specific environmental factors and specific emergencies and threats. We end with navigation and tracking, then the worst case scenario which is bugging out and the hide site.

This book is organized to get you ready for the most common, a mild emergency. Then for moderate. And then extreme. Each layer builds on the other. The key is that you get started and have your base in place.

Tasks/Checklists:
There are numerous tasks/checklists throughout this book. They are marked by the Special Forces patch. Here's a guide to how they are laid out and how to use them:

They are numbered and repeated in Appendix A. Most are labeled either Mild, Mod/Ex (Moderate/Extreme) or

Moderate or Extreme so you can focus on the level you want to accomplish.

Where you see the Ranger tab these are interesting tidbits.

An important aspect we also focus on is the days after an emergency. Since you have water in place now, the most important commodity, you're already ahead of the preparation curve! Think about when you watch the news in the aftermath of any emergency or natural disaster. The first thing being brought in is water.

You've already got your supply.

After all, when word of a pending emergency is announced (and often they come unannounced!), we see unprepared people panicking. There are mobs in stores fighting over a bottle of water and bare shelves. You don't want to be caught up in that. You want to spend your time preparing inside your home, with the supplies needed already on hand.

WHY LISTEN TO ME?

If a disaster struck, who would you want at your side, helping you? A doctor? Lawyer? Policeman? Teacher? While they all have special skills, I submit that the overwhelming choice would be a Special Forces Green Beret. Someone trained in survival, medicine, weapons, tactics, communication, engineering, counter-terrorism, tactical and strategic intelligence and with the capability to be a force multiplier. This last one is key. Another way this book is unique is because your goal should be to plan for dealing with emergencies with a team/family, not a lonely individual holed up in a bunker deep in the hills.

I was part of the committee at the JFK Special Warfare Center and School that revamped the Qualification Course and made SERE (Survival, Evasion, Resistance and Escape) training an entire, separate block.

This book is a step-by-step guide giving you the tactics and techniques Green Berets use to plan for and train to succeed under the toughest of circumstances; thus they will work in every situation you could find yourself. Don't feel that you have to be a Green Beret to use this book. I'm like most people. I'm not a prepper or a hard-core survivalist. I've been trained and have a lot of experience, but my day to day life is pretty normal. I've prepared just like you need to prepare, but prefer room service over sleeping on the side of a mountain. I'm passing on the key knowledge and experience I have acquired through the mindset of someone living in a non-emergency day-to-day lifestyle.

As I began to research the amount of information out there about survival, I was quickly overwhelmed despite having been extensively trained in this area. Between the books, the videos, the internet and the 'reality' shows, the casual person will get swept under. I'm trying to keep this is as simple as possible and looking at it from the point of view of your 'average' person living in an apartment or house who will have to face situations they are probably not prepared for right now. I prefer to start a fire with a lighter rather than making a bow, then a fireboard, then finding a stick, and using all those to start a fire. Let's keep it simple until it gets hard!

We've seen glimpses of what's coming. The Indian Ocean tsunami; Katrina; 9-11; Haiti; the Japanese quake and subsequent tsunami, Hurricane Sandy, the Louisiana floods, Puerto Rico hurricane recovery, California wildfires and so on. But there are many, lesser, emergencies that are more likely.

A key tenet of success for the Green Beret is to act rather than react. When the disaster strikes, it's too late. The clock is ticking. So let's get prepared!

Task Three
***Mild: If you don't have one, get a first aid kit
for your home.***

Example:
First Aid kit: Adventure Med Kit Weekender:
http://amzn.to/2f3gh4c

PREPARATION

Do Your Area Study

WHAT IS AN AREA STUDY?

An Area Study is simply examining your environment with the perspective of evaluating possible assets and threats so you can properly prepare. An Area Study will allow you to tighten down your preparation and focus on things in order of priority. It's not just the environment but also includes yourself and your team.

You must conduct an Area Study of your Area of Operations (AO). This means studying your home, your work, school, and any other locales where you and people on your A-Team spend a significant amount of time. When taking a trip, you should conduct a travel area study, examining the route you will take, your destination, and your route back.

There are so many cases where a thoughtful Area Study followed up by the appropriate preparations would have saved lives. Preparation is so much better than reacting. Which is what we're doing now.

Area Studies can have non-emergency uses, such as if you're considering moving to a new place. An Area Study can provide valuable decision making data.

Think about it. You live in a tsunami zone. Have you actually driven your evacuation route? How long does it take? Have you figured out the quickest escape route on foot, when an accident caused by terrified people blocks the road or everyone in your neighborhood flees at the same time on the same route creating a traffic jam? You work on the 40th floor of a skyscraper. Do you ever look around and ask yourself: how do I get out of here if the normal means of egress are blocked? While schools run active shooter drills, what about the work place?

You've already begun your Area Study and didn't even realize it by doing Task Two. Some of the core questions are already answered: How close are you to the nearest military base? Nearest police station? Firehouse? Hospital? Do you know where the closest emergency room is? How long it will take to get there? How quickly can an ambulance respond to your location? When my wife and I lived on a winding road that was difficult and confusing to travel, during one medical emergency my wife had to be driven to the nearest largest road to meet an ambulance as it came toward us, saving considerable time and perhaps her life.

You want to examine your environment for a lot of things. What can harm you? What can help you? What can hide you? What are your enabling factors? What are your disabling factors? What is the terrain and how can it help you or hamper you in movement? What are the roads, trails, rail, etc. What effect does your environment have on you? What effect will you have on it?

You don't have to answer these questions right now, but you will soon.

In essence, an Area Study requires you to invest some time and energy on research and to look at your surroundings from a different perspective. It can actually be a fun experience and allow you to see the world around you with a different perspective. Get your A-Team involved because we all look at things a little bit differently.

When my A-Team traveled, my engineers would always be looking at things they saw with a unique perspective. When they saw a bridge, they were mentally calculating how to blow it up. When they saw a stream, they were thinking how to provide a water supply to villagers and irrigation for fields. My weapons men would look at terrain for fields of fire for direct and indirect fire weapons. And cover and concealment for us. As a survivor, you have to look at your environment in terms of what you can use and what can be a threat, what can be scavenged and much more, which requires you to assume a different mindset for a while.

We live in a variety of natural environments. There are also a wide range of human developments from urban to remote rural. Thus one size doesn't fit all.

Doing an Area Study is critical so you can tailor your preparation (and the information in this book) for your specific situation. Some threats are going to be of much more importance for you to prepare for than others. For instance, if you live in Oklahoma, the threat of hurricane is nonexistent (so far), but tornados and earthquakes are likely.

The first step is to start with the most important factor: you and those in your A-Team.

THE MILD AREA STUDY

Purpose. Delineate the area being studied—this applies to your home, your work, and any other locations you will likely be. We'll start with you, your home and then expand outward.

Yourself and Your Team:
What special skills and background do you have? The people on your team?
These include medical, construction, problem solving, military, the list is basically about coping with a mild emergency that isn't life-threatening. The key is to know what you can and can't do, and what those around you can and can't do. Think back to the last emergency experienced—what was the reaction? The answer to this will give a heads up to how one will react in the next emergency. There is no right or wrong answer, but awareness helps.

These skills include medical, military, gardening, hunting, survival training and experience, pilot, boat operation, camping, weapons, cooking, land navigation, swimming, communication (personal and technical) construction, problem solving, fire starting, knot tying, the list goes on and on. Under Mod/Ex we'll talk about team building. Think back to the last crisis encountered. What was the instinctual reaction? Some people can react well others panic. This is a reality that has to be factored into any scenario.

Task Four
Mild: Evaluate & list the following for you and each member of your A-Team.

Name:	
Ability to react in an Emergency:	
Special Skill/Background #1:	
Special Skill/Background #2:	
Special Skill/Background #3:	
Special Skill/Background #4	

Overall physical condition

This includes ability to walk, how much of a pack one could carry, physical disabilities, allergies, medical status, special needs, etc.

Task Five
Mild: Evaluate and list the following for you
and each member of your A-Team.

Name:	
Overall physical condition:	
Medical status:	
Allergies:	
Medications:	
Ability to walk/run:	
Special needs:	
Able to swim?	
Able to drive? Access to a vehicles?	

By looking at these checklists you can see what assets and liabilities you and your A-Team have.

Your Home

When we think survival we picture someone out in the wilderness in a pine tree lean-to, but we spend most of our time in our home and it's easy to overlook what we can do to make that environment safer.

When I research data I find statistics that are all over the place because people can't agree on definitions. Once more, those statistics are variables that differ from home to home, so I won't quote many (those of you with pocket protectors and calculators can google them) but let's do an Area Study for your home in terms of the leading areas of concern.

1.   Falls are a leading cause of injury and death. This is more likely based on the previous part of the Area Study: your personal physical condition. Older people, naturally, are more susceptible to falls and getting injured. One in three people 65 or older will suffer a fall leading to serious injury, if not death.

2.   Poisoning goes in the opposite direction for susceptibility: it is more likely for children to be seriously hurt or killed by ingesting a toxic agent.

3.   Children are also susceptible to choking, suffocation, drowning and scalding. This includes airway obstruction.

4.   Water leads to drowning. Do you have a pool? Water nearby?

5.   Fires and burns have already been covered but you will complete a task checklist for fire prevention in a little bit.

The following task lists the things you should do in order to make your home safer. I'm including it under mild because this affects all of us.

To prevent falls

Clear clutter. Pick things up and put them away. How

many times have we tripped over something that doesn't belong on the floor?

Look at your rugs. Are the edges secured? Are folds flattened? Do they slide? Use tape and rug mats underneath to prevent this.

Bathroom: place grab bars and non-slip maps in all bathrooms. The bathroom is very dangerous because water and soap makes things slippery; and if you do fall you're going to hit something hard like a counter or tile floor. We never land on the fluffy pile of freshly laundered towels, do we?

Lighting: make sure all areas are sufficiently lit, particularly staircases. When we live in a 100 year old house, a back stairwell didn't have a light in it. It also turned near the bottom. We have bought a number of motion sensor, battery powered lights in that stairwell and all over the house. Often we put them just as you enter a room inside the door jam or on the wall, low down. They have been life-savers.

Wear slippers or shoes with rubber soles. I can attest to the danger of just socks on wooden stairs. Never a good combination.

Make your stairs safe. If you have small children or they visit, become an expert at installing childproof gates at the top and bottom of stairs. Have handrails for all stairs. Putting carpeting or a runner on wood stairs can be a life-saver.

Use ladders properly and do not exceed specifications. Always place on solid footing. Have someone hold taller ladders at bottom when in use. Make sure leaning ladders are placed against a solid point.

Task Six
Mild: Fall Prevention Checklist

Clear clutter	
Secure edges of all rugs	
Secure rugs to floors so they don't bunch or slide	
Place grab bars and non-slip mats in bathrooms	
Make sure all stairways and dark areas are adequately lit AMIR motion sensor light: https://amzn.to/2LwlkKY	
Wear slippers or shows with rubber bottoms at all time—no socks only!	
Childproof stairs with gates at top and bottom	
Do all stairs have handrails?	

To prevent poisoning

Label all unmarked liquid containers. If you wonder what's in that old plastic jug, assume it's poison. NEVER use food or drink containers to store hazardous material.

Store cleaning products safely and out of reach of children.

Store medicines securely and out of reach of children.

Put child proof cabinet locks on all doors within reach of children.

Have the poison control phone number posted in your kitchen and on speed dial on your cell phone. 800-222-1222.

Never mix household cleaning products together. Some don't like each other and produce toxic gasses, particularly bleach and ammonia. We are not Walter White. Nor do we want to be.

Never mix medicines together without consulting a doctor or pharmacist. Or call the poison help hotline which is monitored 24 hours a day and can give you advice: 800-222-1222.

Monitor your heaters and fireplaces for CO_2 emissions. Have fireplaces cleaned yearly.

Task Seven
Mild: Poison Prevention Checklist

Completed		
	Post Poison Control Number prominently in Kitchen 800-222-1222	
	Label all unmarked liquid containers	
	Insure all cleaning products are stored out of reach of children	
	Insure all medications are stored out of reach of children	
	Put childproof locks on all reachable cabinets	
	Never mix household cleaning products	
	Never mix medications without approval	
	Monitor all heaters and fireplaces for CO2	
	Have fireplaces cleaned annually	

To prevent choking and suffocation

There's a reason certain toys are designated for certain ages. What a child can put in their mouth, they will put in their mouth. Monitor all toys. Legos and similar sized objects can be deadly.

When putting babies to sleep make sure there is nothing around them that can cause suffocation.

Watch children during meals. Do they know how to chew properly before swallowing? Cut up food for younger children into bite-sized portions. Stay away from hard candy and foods that can obstruct the airway.

Put trash bags and other plastic bags in places where children can't get to them. The same with the plastic bag that comes back from the dry-cleaners.

Secure batteries, particularly button batteries, from children.

Task Eight
Mild: Choking/Suffocation Prevention Checklist

	Keep small toys, items out of reach of toddlers	
	Clear sleeping areas for babies from all possible items that could smother them	
	Keep trash bags and plastic bags out of reach of children	
	Keep batteries, especially button batteries, from children	

To prevent drowning and water-related injuries

Always monitor young children when bathing.

Insure your dishwasher and washing machine are off when done.

Never leave water running when you're not watching it. This is not only for injuries but for home damage (speaking from experience).

Don't use electronics around water, especially the bath.

Keep toilet lids closed.

Pools should be completely enclosed with at least a four-foot high fence and childproof gate.

Never allow children in a pool unsupervised.

Task Nine
Mild: Drowning Prevention Checklist

	Never leave water running when not being watched	
	Always monitor small children while bathing	
	Don't use electronics around water, especially bathtub	
	Keep toilet lids closed	
	Pool must be enclosed by minimum 4 foot high fence with childproof gate	
	Never allow children to swim unsupervised	

To prevent fires and burns

Smoke detectors on every floor and every bedroom. Replace batteries every six months. Test your alarm monthly.

Do not leave the kitchen while the stove is on.

Do not leave burning candles unattended over night or when you are not at home.

Task Ten
Mild: Fire Prevention Checklist

	Smoke detectors in every bedroom	
	Smoke detector on every floor	
	Test smoke detectors every money	
	Replace smoke detector batteries every six months	
	Never leave kitchen while stove is on	
	Never leave candles burning overnight or when not home	

To prevent firearms injuries
Lock firearms up in a secure safe and restrict access.
Use trigger guards.
Never leave a loaded firearm unattended.
Follow all firearm safety rules.

Task Eleven
Mild: Firearm Prevention Checklist

	All firearms must be secured in a locked area	
	Locked trigger guards on all firearms	
	Never leave a loaded firearm unattended	
	Know and follow all firearm safety rules	

Your Immediate Area of Operations
That's a fancy way of saying the area around your home, your work, your school, etc. I cover each of those areas in detail in the section on the places for which to plan. Right now let's do your immediate area.

At HomeFacts you will get a listing of the following which will help: crime rate, environmental hazards, crime stats, drug labs, air quality, radon, UV index, brownfields, registered polluters, tanks and spills, average monthly temperatures, probability of earthquakes, hail, hurricanes and tornadoes; closest airports, FCC towers, fire stations, hospitals and police stations.

Task Twelve
Go to Homefacts http://www.homefacts.com/
and enter your zip code.

Home Facts:

Here is what the Knoxville zip code looks like for natural disasters:

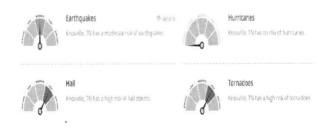

Task Thirteen
Mild: Of the four type of special environments, which ones do you need to be concerned with in order of priority: Cold Weather, Desert, Tropical and Water.

Special Environments
1.
2.
3.

Here is a partial list of natural disasters:

Tornado, Hurricane, Heat Wave, Drought, Wildfire, Blizzard, Earthquake, Tsunami, Volcano, Mud/Landslide, Flooding, Tidal Surge.

Natural Disasters in Order of Likelihood
1.
2.
3.

Below is a partial list of man-made disasters. While some of them are truly accidents and can't be anticipated, others might have a higher likelihood depending on where you live such as a dam failure or industrial accident. Some also depend on your lifestyle such as where you work or whether you own firearms.

Car accident, boat/ferry accident, train/subway accident, tall building evacuation, fire, power outage, burglary, robbery, carjacking, civil unrests/riots, terrorist attack, active shooter, firearms accidents, nuclear power plant accident, nuclear weapons, dam failure, biological weapons and infectious diseases, chemical weapons/accident, industrial accident.

Are your power lines buried? What industries are in your area? What are you downwind, downstream of? What toxic materials and/or gases would be emitted if there was an accident? Where is the closest nuclear power plant or storage area? Are there labs in your area that work with dangerous biological agents? What about the local university? Are you in the flood zone of a dam breaking? Check: http://nid.usace.army.mil/cm_apex/f?p=838:12

For this web site just enter an organization type (any will do) from the drop down menu and you'll be taken to the next page where you can check dams by state. There is also an interactive map.

What rails lines are near you? What is being transported on those lines? Is toxic material being carried? If a train derails and that material is released, what should you do? Under survival, the proper response for a chemical agent is covered—your first instinct to run is usually the wrong one! The same is true for evaluating potential problems on waterways and roads.

Where is your hundred year flood line? You can use the FEMA flood map search to determine this: https://msc.fema.gov/portal/search

Task Fourteen
Mild: Man-made disasters in order of likelihood in your AO

1.
2.
3.
4.
5.

By doing this task, we can now focus on what is important for your specific situation in this manual.

GPS and Maps

A key step in conducting an Area Study is to have maps. Actual, physical maps. We are a society that is overly reliant on technology in many ways. Cell phones for communication are one. GPS for navigating is another.

GPS stands for Global Positioning System. A basic understanding of GPS is useful so we understand what it can do and can't do.

Let's get a little geeky. The GPS receiver gets a signal from each satellite with the exact time it is sent. By subtracting the time the signal was sent from the time it was received the GPS receiver can calculate how far it is from the satellite. The receiver knows where the satellite is in orbit so it has a fix on that satellite. For our GPS receiver to work it needs to make contact and get a fix with at least 3 GPS satellites for a two dimensional fix (latitude and longitude) and 4 satellites for a three dimensional fix (adding in elevation). If you are only getting 3 satellites and aren't at sea level, your actual location could be different from what the GPS is showing. If you're up at a high altitude in the mountains, this can become significant. Usually, though, this isn't a problem. Of the 31 active GPS satellites, there are usually 6 in range from most places on the Earth's surface.

Ever notice that it takes your GPS varying amounts of time to get a fix? If the GPS hasn't been on recently it could take as long as 30 seconds. Tall buildings or other obstructions can also make it take longer. Most GPS accuracy is to within 5 meters.

Cellphone GPS units act a bit differently incorporating Assisted-GPS to get a fix quickly. They use cell phone tower data to assist. Sometimes they can give you a fix without even accessing satellites. This only works though it you are in cellphone and Wifi coverage. Outside of that, you're out of luck.

Another thing to consider is whether the map coverage you're using is in your device's memory or downloading. Ever have the map become blank when you're out of coverage? We should always download our local area tiles for whatever mapping GPS we use. When I plan trips, I download the map tiles into memory for the route and destination. This allows the GPS to work faster and gives me a map even if I can't download it live. For your vehicle's GPS are the maps you're using in the memory or downloading? Put them in the memory.

I've noticed when biking and using GPS that every so often it will tell me it has lost the signal. Some of these 'dead spots' are the same, but others seem random. Which brings me to this significant point: you can't count on GPS!

There are other problems with GPS:

They rely on the satellites working. EMP—electromagnetic pulse, whether natural (solar flare) or man-made (nuclear weapon) can wipe those satellites out.

The GPS receiver, whether in your vehicle, a cell phone or handheld GPS receiver, requires power to work. Cell phones and batteries can die. Commercial airplanes are required to have backup navigation to GPS. Just in case. We need to do the same.

Sadly, many people no longer carry paper maps in their car. Beyond that, many don't know how to read a road map, never mind a topographical one.

When I was a brand new butter-bar second lieutenant in the First Cavalry Division, I was told succinctly that a platoon leader had to do two things well: Maintain communications on the radio and navigate. Failing either of those two and your time as leader was limited and your career in the Army over.

In a survival situation, especially moderate to extreme, it is highly likely you will have to move from point A to point B. It also possible you won't have a GPS to do that with.

Have a road map as a backup. I keep a Rand McNally binder with maps of North America inside my Jeep.

It gets used so much (even when I have GPS because I like to wander) that I buy a new one every year because a few heavily perused pages get worn out and torn, not that I'm blaming Cool Gus who sometimes sits on it in the passenger seat, but I'm blaming Cool Gus.

While Rand McNally is great for your car, get topographic maps of your locale. The scale you want for local area is 1:24,000. You can download and print out maps at this scale for free from the sites below. You can also buy a large map book of your state with topographic maps.

For the National Geographic maps it's pretty cool because you can download the maps in sets of five where the first is an overview of the quadrant, then the other four are printer sized. Print out in color!

You can also get maps from USGS. These maps allow you to pick the details you want. Also, you can get different scales. 7.5 minute is 1:24,000. Which means one inch on the map equals 24,000 inches on the ground or 2000 feet. 15 minutes is 1:63,360.

Task Fifteen Mild: GPS/Map Checklist

	Road atlas for each car. Rand McNally Road Atlas. https://amzn.to/2LwlO3B	
	Download or buy topographic maps for your area of operation: National Geographic Maps: http://www.natgeomaps.com/trail-maps/pdf-quads USGS Maps: http://nationalmap.gov/ustopo/	
	Get a waterproof map case to put your top maps in, with dummy cord. Waterproof map case. https://amzn.to/2BBhaNm	
	Get a topographic atlas of your area DeLorme Tennessee Atlas & Gazetteer: https://amzn.to/2BBhwna	
	Download the map tiles for your area of operation for your car GPS (if possible), your phone, and handheld GPS (if used)	

The topographic maps should include your immediate area. If you believe you are going to have to evacuate, get maps covering the route and your BOHS. Then get a waterproof map case.

Then get a dummy cord (a piece of 550 cord works fine) to tie the map off to you. The one above already comes with a cord. Seriously. I can't tell you how many times that dummy cord kept me from being stupid and losing my map.

You can order laminated, waterproofed maps, but they are more difficult to carry because of limited folding. This is a judgment call on your part. I prefer the paper map inside of a waterproof map case. For geeks, you can get a pocket protector and alcohol pens to write on the case and the special eraser for the writing when you're done drawing and then . . .

You can order topographic maps by states. I keep this in my Jeep to back up my road map. You can also go to your local camping store or local bookstore and you should be able to get the pertinent sets of maps. Land Navigation is covered in Survival.

Feeling a bit overwhelmed? Here's the easy way to do it. Start from your house. Then move outwards. Do the same with your work. Look at the route from home to work/school. And your Emergency Rally Point. And BOHS. A lot of the information will overlap.

Check one thing at a time. Write down your observations. You'll be surprised at the amount of information you end up with and how much wiser and mentally prepared you will be than you were. Make sure you 'disseminate the information' to your A-Team. Actually, what's best is if you break down the Area Study and have different members of the team do different parts. Then brief each other. This can actually be an enlightening and fun exercise.

Once you have the Area Study done, adjust your planning and preparedness to fit the order of likelihood of emergencies and disasters.

EMERGENCY RALLY POINT (ERP) AND APPS

Before we discuss the ERP, we need to consider when you would use it. The most likely scenario is if there is an event where you can't get to your home or to the IRP near your home. A flood, wildfire, earthquake, etc. could cause this.

Thus you need a location where your A-Team will meet. This place is where they will automatically go even if there is no communication. After major disasters, many people rue that they didn't have such a spot picked out because they spent many hours and even days separated and wondering about each other's status.

There are no hard and fast rules when you should utilize the ERP. Every situation is going to be different. The key is at the very least choose the ERP and make sure everyone knows where it is. It cannot be picked after the emergency has begun.

You can choose the house of a friend/relative that is out of the immediate area of your home. Someone's school or work place.

Choose the ERP based on the Area Study you've just done. If your most likely threat is tsunami, you'd pick an ERP out of range of that event. The same with a flood. It should be out of the range of the most likely threats, yet a point where everyone in your A-Tcam can get to.

There are apps that can be used to help locate family members; however, like every other thing associated with your cell phone they require power, cell coverage, etc. Be sure to make sure these apps work and that they are installed on all phones. Be aware that some can be heavy draws on battery life if active. Each has pros and cons so do a little research. I use Road ID on a daily basis when out biking or kayaking, just in case. I like that it will send a notification to my emergency contact if I am stationery for more than a designated period or pass an overall time limit, along with tracking my location.

A WORD ON USING APPS!
Don't just download an App and ignore. Open it. Most require some form of sign in which could be awkward during an emergency.
Explore it. How does it work? What does it do and what doesn't it do?
Some apps are battery intensive, especially locator apps.
You can never rely 100% on any app because they are dependent on your phone which is dependent on:
-You having your phone
-The phone working
-the battery
-often apps require getting a signal

Task Sixteen
Mild: Download Locator Apps

Road ID Here is their home page with links to both Apple and Android along with information on how the app works. https://www.roadid.com/pages/road-id-app	
Life 360 Android: https://play.google.com/store/apps/details?id=com.life360.android.safetymapd Apple: https://itunes.apple.com/us/app/life360-family-tracker/id384830320?mt=8	
Sygic Family locator Android: https://play.google.com/store/apps/details?id=com.sygic.familywhere.android&hl=cs&referrer=utm_source%3Dsygic-com%26utm_medium%3Dheader-features%26utm_campaign%3Dfamily-locator Apple: https://itunes.apple.com/sk/app/family-locator-gps-tracker/id588364107?mt=8	
Trusted Contacts: Android: https://play.google.com/store/apps/details?id=com.google.android.apps.emergencyassist&utm_source=google&utm_medium=web&utm_campaign=homepage Apple: https://itunes.apple.com/app/trusted-contacts/id1225684042	

You use the ERP in conjunction with your out of state emergency contact.

THE MODERATE/EXTREME (MOD/EX) AREA STUDY

This is basically studying the environment around you in more detail, but with an eye to what it would be like to traverse it (whether by car, foot, boat, etc) and survive in it.

Climate: Note variations from the norm and the months in which they occur. Note any extremes in climate.

Temperature: Know the extremes and norms. If you've lived somewhere for several years, you probably have a good feel for this. However, if you are new to an area, take some time to study up.

Rainfall and snow: This is a good news, bad news area. The good news is rainfall and snow provide water. The bad news is they can make shelter difficult. They can also lead to hypothermia.

Seasonal effect of weather: There are places where weather can change drastically in just a day. When we lived in Colorado there was a saying: If you don't like the weather, just wait. It will be different in a couple of days. It's not just seasonal, also consider altitude.

Elevation and Temperature
It's a rule of thumb that on a sunny day every 1,000 feet gained in altitude means a drop in temperature of

5.4 degrees Fahrenheit and on a cloudy day 3.3 degrees Fahrenheit.

Every year several hikers die on Mount Washington in the summer because they start out in short and t-shirts with no cold weather gear and freeze to death before they reach the summit after getting caught in a storm that also reduces visibility to almost nothing and they lose the trail.

Terrain: General direction of mountain ranges or ridgelines. If you are traveling, have an idea of the terrain you are going through, especially if it is different from what you are used to. General degree of slope. Considering your physical condition, and that of members of your team, what can you climb and descend?

Characteristics of valleys and plains. What directions do the valleys run?

Natural routes for and natural obstacles to cross-country movement. When we lived on Whidbey Island, it fascinated us how isolated the city of Seattle is by land. There are only a handful of roads into the Seattle area, particularly from the east through the Cascades. And even to the south, coming up from Oregon, your routes are limited. The same is true for Los Angeles and San Diego, where the San Andreas fault and the mountains are to the east and could easily isolate those areas by land. Look at where you live and check your area for your choke points.

Overall region: mountainous, prairie, mountains, coastal, swamp, etc: If you live in a forested area, have you ever tried moving cross-country in it? After doing survival training in the deep woods of Maine, one can easily understand why Stephen King writes horror. It is almost impossible to travel through some forests in Maine. A woman recently died after getting off the Appalachian Trail in Maine and was unable to find the trail again. The same is true of the Pacific Northwest. The first time you try moving through nature shouldn't be the survival situation. Get off the path and see how tough the going is in the land around you.

Rivers and streams; Bridges, other crossing points; main rivers and direction of flow. What is downstream? What is upstream?

For rivers and streams, understand the water system. What is the natural water drainage system in your area? This can help in determining location and direction.

Rivers can be a route of transportation or an obstacle. During one mission my team had to cross a glacial river. We knew the water would be just above freezing so we carried a dry suit with us so the lead scout could swim a line across the river and we could build a rope bridge. When we got to the river we saw a large animal (bigger than us) swept away by the current. Change in plans. We ended up crossing the river by using the girders underneath the bridge at night with security on high ground using night vision goggles to watch for traffic.

What rivers and streams are in your area? If you have to cross them, how will you? Remember, bridges are choke points. In extreme emergencies expect unsavory elements to use this to their advantage.

Characteristics of rivers and streams, including widths, currents, banks, depths, kinds of bottoms, and obstacles. Note seasonal variations, such as dry beds, flash floods. A creek can turn into a raging torrent in the spring when the snow pack melts. The Tennessee River drops in the winter as the TVA lowers the water level via dams to prevent flooding. While obvious in retrospect I researched why and the answer is simple: in winter the vegetation does not absorb as much water as in summer, thus flooding can occur quicker.

If on a river, what is downstream? Upstream?

Lakes, ponds, swamps: What lakes, ponds and

swamps are in your area? These kinds of areas can be very difficult to move through. However, that also makes them a great area to hide in. Think of what Francis Marion, the "Swamp Fox" was able to achieve during the Revolutionary War in the low country of South Carolina.

Coastline: Learn about tides and waves along with the effect of wind and current. We'll cover this in more detail in special environments, but many people have lost their lives not understanding the local tides and the power of tidal surge during a storm.

Water is extraordinarily powerful. You cannot defeat it. Hurricane Sandy caused so much devastation because it was a combination of the storm and the tide. When I lived on the Intracoastal Waterway in South Carolina it was amazing to see the difference between a high-high tide and a low-low tide. When a storm hits in concert with high tide, that's a worst-case scenario.

Water is powerful! During maritime operations training, we camped on a lighthouse island off the coast of Maine for several weeks as our base of operations. My team sergeant, experienced in water operations, had us swim landward into the mouth of a river, while the tide was going out, to teach us a lesson. No matter how hard we finned, we went seaward.

Primary Roads: What are the primary roads in your area? Assume these will be clogged in a moderate or extreme emergency.

Secondary Roads: Are there ways to get out of the area using backroads that people will be less likely to take?

Natural routes on foot: If you have to bug out, what route will you take?

Evacuation routes: Do you know your hurricane evacuation route? Your tsunami evacuation route? More on this under those specific topics in Survival.

Rail lines: What rails lines are near you? What is being transported on those lines? Is toxic material being carried? If a train derails and that material is released, what should you do? Are there abandoned rail lines in your AO? Rail lines, whether in use or abandoned can often be excellent on-foot escape routes. Knowing the rail lines can also help in navigation and orientation.

Water sources: Note ground, surface, seasonal, and potable. Find the closest natural source of water to your home, work and ERP. Assume it needs to be purified. Does it flow year round?

Food sources: Seasonal or year-round.
Cultivated. Include vegetables, grains, fruits, and nuts. What farms are in your area? What crops do they raise?
Natural. Include berries, fruits, nuts, and herbs. What is edible in your environment?
Domesticated animals in the area. Aka, a food source. What is around you?
Wildlife. Include animals, fish, and fowl.

YOUR SURVIVAL A-TEAM

Mild A-Team
For many of us, a 'team' is a no-brainer'. Our family is our survival team. For others, though, this is a decision: whether to try to make it on their own or join forces with others. There are advantages and disadvantages to a team, which also change depending on whether you have a mild, moderate or extreme emergency. Here are some for you to consider:

Advantages
The whole is greater than the sum of its parts. You can't be an expert on everything. Having an array of people who bring different, needed skills, is important. Some people just can't handle being alone. Can you?

A sense of purpose. In combat, soldiers fight for each other, not for a cause. Being a member of a team can increase your motivation to get out of yourself and fight for the survival of those who you care about and are with you.

In an extreme emergency, long term survival will eventually depend on team building. In this scenario you often won't have much of a choice who you will ally with. Groups will form with different agendas. You have to evaluate your goals, and also whether you will be an asset to the team. What do you bring to the table?

Disadvantages
You make a larger target. It is indeed better to run away rather than fight. Your running away is limited by your slowest member. The only soldier I had to remove my A-Team couldn't keep up with us in the field, carrying our

extremely heavy combat load. You are also more likely to be discovered in an extreme survival situation as part of a team.

You are letting others in on your survival plan. The lazy survivalist simply lets others prepare, then comes in and plunders.

Will the other members of the team be prepared? If it's your family, it's your responsibility to get them ready since you're reading this.

Will the members of the team actually pull their weight? To wait until a survival situation to evaluate team-members is foolhardy. Security gets looser, the more people on the team. I call it the trust ripple effect. How many people do you trust? Trust with your life? How many people do they trust? In the move *Contagion*, as soon as the CDC character tells his wife about the outbreak and to get out of town, warning her to 'TELL NO ONE', what does she immediately do? Tell someone. As Ben Franklin said: "Three may keep a secret, if two of them are dead." In covert operations we tended to be very paranoid, but you're not paranoid if they are out to get you.

Where to find survival A-Team members?
Most likely it will be your family.

Think about last Thanksgiving. Do you really want to huddle in a hide site with those people?

Joking.

Not.

In mild to moderate emergencies, you will want to gather your family and team members as quickly as possible.

Other places to find potential survival buddies:
Your friends.

From your job. Actually, you should quietly evaluate your co-workers anyway, because the percentage of time you spend at work is the percentage chance an emergency or natural disaster will strike while you are among them. On 9-11 certain co-workers proved to be true life-savers.

Your church

Hunting and garden clubs. Two extremes here, but each brings something to the table.

Those attending self-defense classes or survival workshops.

Organizing Your Neighborhood/Work Place

This is particularly key in moderate emergencies. During natural disasters such as hurricane, flood, extreme weather, wild fire, etc. an organized neighborhood can be essential to survival. When I say neighborhood, I also mean your work place. On Nine-Eleven, offices in the World Trade Center that were well organized and had emergency evacuation plans with designated personnel acting in key positions had much higher survival rates. Does your place of business have an emergency plan? Is it practiced? Remember in school when you had fire drills? Does your place of business have the same?

One thing to ask yourself is what are the boundaries of a neighborhood? Realistically, you're looking at around fifteen to twenty households. Larger than that and it can become unwieldy.

Your neighborhood might already have such a team. If so, join it and find out how well organized and prepared they are. If not, then take it on yourself to start one. Usually your larger community will have resources to help you do this. Contact emergency services and the Red Cross and ask.

Do you know who your neighbors are and what they do for a living? What special skills they have? That person you think is a nurse going off to work in her scrubs might actually be someone who works at a kennel washing dogs. Don't make assumptions.

Inventory the neighborhood:
Chain saws
Winches
Four wheel drive vehicles
CB and other radios
Water purifying systems
Where are all the natural gas meters and propane tanks?

Who needs special help? Focus on the handicapped, the elderly, and children who might be home alone at periods of the day.

Each household should have large placards made up with OKAY on one side and HELP on the other. Use fluorescent colored poster board available at your local supermarket. Have this stored near a front window under a rug. Display as needed.

Determine where the neighborhood gathering site will be. People should go here before trying to run around and rescue others. Organization saves time and lives.

Have a contact list tree of who alerts who. In the military we always had alert systems. This is a way of communicating so each person knows who they are responsible for contacting.

Preparing the physically challenged
Keep on you a list of all medications, allergies, special equipment, along with the names and contact information of doctors, pharmacists and family members.

Keep extra medications on hand.

Keep emergency supplies within reach and if in a wheelchair, have a way to take them with you.

Have a whistle to signal for help.

During an emergency situation, have at least two people who you can count on to check on you. Make sure they know your special needs, how to operate any special equipment, what meds you take and the schedule, and where your emergency supplies are.

If you evacuate your home, leave a message so those two people checking on you know you've left and where you are going.

Preparing the Elderly
Keep walking aids close by at all times.

Have extra medications on hand.

Put a security light in every room. These plug in and automatically go on if there is a loss of electricity.

Have a whistle on hand.

Have at least two people who will check on you.

Pets
Yes, they actually sell pet survival kits. You laugh. You won't if you need to evacuate.

The key to pet survival is what is good for you, is good for them: water, food, and shelter being key.

If you evacuate, do not leave your pets behind. However, if you are going to a public shelter, understand that pets might not be allowed inside. Do you have an alternative for them? Check hotels in the area to which you will evacuate and find which ones will accept pets under those conditions. Check with your local animal shelter and get their advice. At the absolute very least, set them free.

Take pet food, bottled water, medications (tick and heartworm meds), vet records, cat litter/pan, can opener, food dishes, water dishes, and any other supplies as needed. We use a large plastic container for our dog food and store the dishes and all their supplies inside, on top of the food. Keeping everything in one place makes it easy to grab it and go if needed.

Make sure your pet id tags are up to date with your current cell phone number and address. If evacuating, attach the evac destination on their collar with paper covered with clear tape or a label maker.

Make sure you have a current photo of your pet for identification purposes.

Make sure you have a leash and collar to control your pet.

Mild Team Communication

We rely on cell phones and the point has been made that they might be not be reliable.

One thing to remember is that a text message has a greater chance of getting through than voice if the cell phone system is overwhelmed after a wide-spread disaster.

Land-lines have fallen out of favor with many people, but there are times a land-line will work when cells won't. However, it is also reliant on the system to be intact.

The Internet is another common mode of information, but less reliable than cell phones since it requires both power and a connection. Of course, it's reliant on the system being viable. Twitter is an excellent early-warning system with live reporting. However, also be aware that the Internet is often full of bogus material.

Two-way radios are an option for an A-Team. Because they are FM, their range is limited. They are also half-duplex, which means you have one channel so you are either transmitting or receiving. Thus the use of the term 'Over' when you are done transmitting and release the transmit button. (For picky people, you never say 'over and out' because 'over' means you are awaiting a response and 'out' means you're done and not expecting a response).

Most decent two-way FM radios have a range of about two-miles but buildings and terrain can limit that as FM waves travel in straight lines.

There are other two way radios that claim much longer ranges using GMRS (General Mobile Radio Service) which is basically what CBs use. The issue with all these radios is battery life.

Mod/Ex A-TEAM

Let's briefly discuss a team that already exists and is the perfect combination for a survival situation: the Special Forces A-Team. Reviewing the specialties on an A-Team can give you a good idea of the ideal survival team. While bearing in mind that the A-Team is built for war, an extreme situation will involve war-like conditions.

The A-Team

The A-Team is the operational element of Special Forces. It is designed to conduct operations completely on its own, unlike the rest of the army, which has a hierarchy of tactical and strategic operations. In a survival situation, your team must be able to operate on its own, without any external support.

An A-Team consists of twelve people as follows (note the array of essential skills):

Team Leader

A captain who exercises command of the detachment. Your survival team must have a designated leader who can make decisions while under great stress and experiencing uncertainty. This ability to make decisions trumps all other traits.

Team Sergeant

Officially known as the Operations Sergeant and the senior enlisted member of the detachment. He advises the team leader on operations and training matters. He provides tactical and technical guidance and professional support to detachment members.

For your team, while the team leader looks to the outside world, the team sergeant looks to the welfare of the people on the team. Combining two people who can work together, one focusing outward and one focusing inward, and you can have an extremely effective team.

Executive Officer

Officially known as the detachment technician. Serves as second in command and ensures that the detachment commander's decisions and concepts are implemented. He prepares the administrative and logistical portions of area studies, briefbacks and OPLANs.

This is the person who replaces the team leader as needed. Also, if you have to split your team up, the XO commands the second part.

The Assistant Operations and Intelligence Sergeant

Plans, coordinates and directs the detachment's intelligence collections, analysis, production and dissemination. He also assists the Operations Sergeant and replaces him when needed. This is the person who should be most up to speed on the area study and focuses on the current situation and projects out possibilities.

Two Weapons Sergeants

They train detachments members and indigenous personnel in the use of individual small arms, light crew-served weapons and anti-air and anti-armor weapons.

Who are your weapon experts? Both conventional and expedient? Can they train other team members to proficiency if need be? Do you have people experienced in hunting on your team?

Two Engineer Sergeants

Supervise, lead, plan, perform and instruct all aspects of combat engineering and light construction engineering.

They construct and employ improvised munitions. They plan and perform sabotage operations.

Who are your handy-men/women? People who've worked construction? Also, consider those who are gardeners and know how to grow food. These people are indispensable in an extreme emergency.

Two Medical Sergeants

Provide emergency, routine, and long-term medical care for detachment members and associated allied or indigenous personnel. They establish medical facilities to support detachment operations.

Some of the most valuable people in a survival situation are medical personnel. Recruiting someone with medical training should be a high priority. Think outside the norm here. EMTs, veterinarians, midwives, witches, former military medics, etc.

Two Communications Sergeants

Install, operate, and maintain FM, AM, HF, VHF, UHF and SHF radio communications in voice, CW, and burst radio nets. Who is going to be in charge of your link to the rest of the world? Who will maintain and monitor communications? Who's the geek on the team?

You're seeing a pattern. Find what training, experience, hobbies, etc. people have. Success in survival isn't necessarily equal to success in civilization. The ability to sew during the Andes plane crash incident was a life-saver. This was chronicles in the book *Alive!*. I cover the sequence of events during this in *Stuff Doesn't Just Happen II: The Gift of Failure*.

Who Do You Want On your A-Team?

Often this won't be a choice. You're going with your family/loved ones.

However there are those who want to build a team and/or train their family members/loved ones in the necessary skills for a survival team.

Using the A-Team above, let's discuss who you'd want to have on your team and what skills they should have before an emergency. These are also the choices you might have to make while in an or after an extreme emergency/catastrophe.

The first person many think of is someone who is ex-military. I even point out that you'd most likely want a Green Beret as your #1 choice, but remember, those are Special Forces; not your run of the mill military person. The majority of veterans, while they have some basic training, were support personnel, so you have to consider what their MOS- military occupation specialty—was.

Then there is the 'prepper'. Unfortunately, too many people confuse owning a bunch of guns and stockpiling ammunition and food as 'preparing'. As you can see from this manual, I give little mention to this topic. First, if firing guns comes into play, you are in, or just escalated into, an extreme emergency. The odds of a mild or moderate emergency are much, much higher and need to be prepared for first.

Simply owning guns, doesn't mean a person knows how to use them. Even hunters who use long guns may be great shots, but there's a big difference when we're talking Close Quarters Battle.

The other issue with guns is you can only carry a couple. Unless you're a "shooter", someone whose full time job is training on weapons, you can only be proficient on a couple of guns. It's better to have two you know how to use than 40 sitting in your gun locker.

So who do you want?

The most important attribute is someone who handles crisis well. Who doesn't panic. Unless you've actually seen someone in an emergency, this is a hard quality to ascertain.

Focus on skill sets:

Medical

Law enforcement and military

Leadership

Survival

Communications

Engineering

Weapons (both close quarters battle and hunting)

Gardening, farming

Ranching

Electrical

Scavenging. This last one is a skill one rarely thinks of. But as we will see in Survival, a key phase after a moderate to extreme emergency is scavenging. Not just scavenging (being able to find things), but also the ability to improvise. A MacGyver type of person, who can make something out of disparate parts. Who can find different uses for things. Interestingly, often woman are better at this than men because men tend to be linear thinkers. For a man the only way to get to B is from A. Women tend to be circular thinkers and they might think the best way to get to B from A, is to go to C and loop back.

Team-Building

To truly bring a team together, a variation of something that we developed in the 2d Battalion, 10th Special Forces Group (Airborne), can be very useful: gut checks.

It would be worthwhile to perform some sort of gut check with those you plan on being on your extreme survival team. There are even civilian "tests" like Tough Mudder that "push" you under difficult circumstances. Remember one thing though: they do not have the added stressor of life or death. That can completely change even the toughest "mudder" into the biggest loser.

The core intent of a gut check, in whatever format you come up with, is to put individuals and teams in crisis. When I consulted with a nursing department at a major university, their form of the gut check was to run a mass casualty simulation for the students. This was a moderate emergency for them, which they practiced regularly.

A person's true nature comes out during a crisis. In the same manner the strengths and weaknesses of a team can quickly be determined.

A key decision that has to be made beforehand is a chain of command. Someone must be the leader. And so on, down to the last person, the minion, because every team needs a minion. Remember that survival leadership requires different traits than normal, civilian leadership. A key trait is the ability to make decisions while in crisis.

A survival group is not a democracy. Often there is no time to sit around and debate options. Decisions have to be made quickly. Hammer out the leadership issue before the emergency.

Mod/Ex Team Communication

It is unlikely your team will all be in the same place when a disaster strikes. We are overly reliant on cell phone communication. In a moderate or extreme emergency, it is likely that this service will either be interrupted (lack of power, towers destroyed) or overwhelmed with too many people trying to call at the same time. On 9-11, many people were frustrated in their attempts to use their cell phones.

Also, if there is an extended power outage, even if service isn't interrupted, will you be able to recharge your cell phones?

When you consider using a GPS on your cell phone, remember that in many cases, the mapping information is being downloaded from your net if you haven't already downloaded it into the memory. Thus if your service is interrupted, your cell phone GPS can tell you where you are, but it might not display the map. Understand that the GPS on your cell (and many apps) are a way you can be tracked by people who have access to the technology. Most people don't understand that they are basically carrying a tracking device with them all the time (their cell phone). It's also a listening device.

There are other options.

GMRS and FRS radios work well for short distances, but their range is limited. If you are interested in learning about radio waves, etc. go to another source. Suffice it to say, that any system you use, make sure you test it. A problem with these systems is they require power to work. These usually work line of sight. So while the manufacturer might state they work 30-40 miles, the reality is, in uneven terrain, their effectiveness will be more limited. If purchasing these types of radios, get ones that run on 12 volt DC or rechargeable battery packs. It helps if they can also run on conventional batteries as you should have a supply of those on hand.

CB radios are also an option, with greater range. Again, power consumption is a problem. Also, no matter what system you use, remember that anyone can be listening in on your frequency or channel. If you don't live near water that people boat on, a sneaky way to communicate can be to get VDC marine radios. The bottom line, however, is assume any transmission you make is being listened to by others in an extreme emergency. So don't be broadcasting to a team member "oh my gosh, we have so much food here, we don't know what to do with it. Hurry up and join us for the feast tonight." You might end up with too many dinner guests.

In Special Forces we encrypted all our transmissions. The easiest way for your team is to have a short list of code words that mean various things.

Task Seventeen Mod/Ex: A-Team Code Word

Word/Phrase	Code Word
Home	
IRP	
ERP	
HIDE SITE	
I've been compromised and am sending this under duress.	
Code name for team member #1:	
Code name for team member #2:	
Code name for team member #3:	
Code name for team member #4:	
Code name for team member #5:	
Code name for team member #6:	
Code word for every day of week.	
Anchor Point for team	
Add whatever key words you believe you need	

The key is if your code word for your ERP is Orange, if you say "let's meet at Orange" no one else will know where you're talking about. If you say "Orange is compromised", the same thing. Your team mates know not to go to the ERP.

A system for days of the week and how many weeks. This allows you to coordinate a link up. If you sit for a few minutes and talk it out with team members, you will quickly realize there is a bunch of information you would want to transmit back and forth without someone understanding exactly what you're saying. Make up your lists accordingly.

The Anchor Point is a spot you can use to communicate locations securely as long as no one else knows it: You can transmit: *I am three-point-five kilometers from (code word for Anchor Point) at an azimuth of 127 degrees.*

Not only do code words make your communication more secure, they can also shorten your transmission time, which is always a plus as it saves power.

Pick two times a day to make communication. Much like Will Smith in *I Am Legend*, pick a certain time when members on your team will know your system is on. This allows you to save battery life. It also allows you to focus on other things, rather than hanging around the cell phone or radio all day.

In Special Forces we had two communications sergeants on each A-Team, an indication of how valuable we viewed this skill. While we are now overly reliant on satellite communications, these men are trained on other types of radios, including high frequency. A local Ham radio operator would be a good person to get to know. They might end up being the only one getting information from the "outside" world. There is something that can seriously disrupt communications. Electromagnetic Pulse, better known as EMP, is a high-intensity burst of electromagnetic particles. I discuss this further on, under Solar Flare.

Other Team Considerations

Your primary team shelter will be a home. Pick the one that is most amendable to the survival requirements as laid out in this book.

You should have a team IRP, ERP and BOHS.

Briefly the BOHS Site is where everyone will link up once the aliens blow up the White House, the Empire State Building and the local Home Depot. Seriously it is where the team will meet if the IRP and ERP are not viable. This is where you team gathers when things have hit the fan. The key to this Hide Site is it must be located in a hidden and relatively secure location. You must be able to put surveillance on this spot, so that if a team member is coerced into leading someone to this spot, you can see them, before they see you.

Normally in covert operations when making a personal meeting, you would have a safe signal. However, in a survival situation, you don't know who the first person arriving at the ERP will be. What you need is a danger signal. A signal that someone who is coerced to give up the location and leads the bad guys to it, will either emplace or remove so that others coming to the site will see in place, or not in place, whichever is decided upon, and know it's not safe to approach.

Feeling James Bondish? This is all basic tradecraft that was learned in covert operations via what I call blood lessons—people dying. Practice meeting up at your IRP and ERP and BOHS at least once.

Preparing your A-Team

Besides all the equipment and planning preparation listed in this book, you should also conduct rehearsals as needed. At the very least, rehearse assembling at your IRP and ERP. Make sure everyone knows exactly where these are. Make sure they understand the route and an alternate route.

If you have children, get the daycare or school's emergency SOP and find out how they will act in time of crisis. Have plans for someone to pick up your children if you can't make it. Schools have SOPs for many different events and you should have a copy of it. Coordinate an IRP near the school with your child.

If someone on your A-Team doesn't speak English, have a card in English made up with that person's name, address and any special needs, such as medications or allergies.

Make sure everyone knows the safe room and the safest place in each room in the house.

Make sure everyone knows where the shut off for gas, electricity and water are located.

Keep copies of all vital records in your fireproof lockbox.

Cribs should be clear of windows that could implode and heavy furniture that might fall over.

While you've baby-proofed your house for your toddler, putting latches on all the cabinets he/she can reach, what happens during an explosion or earthquakes if higher cabinets come open and spill contents? Consider latching those too.

Make sure your children know what gas and propane smell like.

We now move on to the five key elements of survival.

Task Eighteen
Mild: If you don't have one, get an emergency
radio for your home.

Example:
Survival radio: https://amzn.to/2BBBaiN

Prepare the Five Key Elements For Survival

Congratulations. You now have the three most important items needed for preparation!

We take most of the five key elements for granted, and one of them we rarely think about, but consider how important the following are:

Water
Food
First Aid
Shelter
Fire

WATER

You already have an adequate supply of emergency water in your home based on the first thing in this book you did: get enough water for mild preparation.

Let's talk about water a little more, why it's so important, and what else you need to prepare about it. In our normal lives acquiring water is relatively easy. Turn on the tap to get drinkable water. While many people focus on the power going out, of more essence to survival is the loss of potable water. Your water depends on a source, power and pipes, all of which can be disrupted by a wide array of emergencies. How much drinkable water do you have on hand without relying on the tap?

Another huge factor for water availability is when your normal water source gets contaminated. This is becoming more and more common. Flint, Michigan is an example of long term contamination. But one of the by-products of floods is that the water supply quickly gets polluted as contaminants in the ground and in various storage facilities are mixed together with the flooding waters. If you watch disaster relief, the first thing that is brought in is potable water. Eighty percent of natural disasters are accompanied by flood.

I recommend for Mod/Ex getting a water filter. We always put a high end water filter in any house we live in, preferably whole house, but at least for the sink which is where get our drinking water and store in metal drinking containers. A portable filter is great for emergencies.

Separate from the normal sources of water in civilization, do you know how to acquire safe, drinkable, water? Do you have a source of water within reasonable distance of where you live? Is the water drinkable? Can you make it drinkable? You have to assume that any water that is not marked as potable (drinkable) is contaminated. Even in the deepest forest, there is a chance the water is tainted. Always stay on the safe side, because contracting giardia is no fun at all and cholera can be fatal.

On average, we can survive three days without water versus three weeks without food.

Over three-quarters of your body is composed of fluid. Perspiration is not the only way you lose water. We actually lose more water just by breathing. And you can't stop *that* loss. We lose around 2 to 4 cups of water a day by exhaling (16 cups equal one gallon). We lose about 2 cups via perspiration. We lose ½ to a cup just from the soles of our feet. We lose six cups via urination. When you add that up (and it wasn't easy converting all that) you lose more than half a gallon of water a day just existing; more depending on the weather and your activity level.

Water is critical for functioning. A 5% drop in body fluid will cause a 25% drop in energy level. A 15% drop will cause death. Even in normal day-to-day living, it is estimated that 80% of people are fatigued simply because they are chronically dehydrated.

In your home, you need to be prepared for at least 3 days for mild emergencies, but I recommend doubling that. Your average water bottle is 500 milliliter. Here's the math to make it easy: 7.5 bottles equal a gallon. Your average case of water has 24 bottles, so let's round up to three gallons. That will last a person 3 days. A case of water per person in the household will last three days. If you are in a very hot environment, definitely double that.

Regardless, I recommend storing at the very least *two cases of water per person in the household.* The FDA considers bottled water to have no expiration date as long as the lid is sealed. Expiration dates printed on bottles are voluntary and reflect concern over taste and color; not safety.

Depending on the possibilities of emergencies in your area, more is better. FEMA recommends having at least a two-week supply for moderate emergencies. I recommend a month at a gallon per person, per day for extreme emergencies.

***This is your number one priority: Get the water if
you haven't already!
Stop procrastinating.***

In your home, you can add another half-gallon of water
per person for things such as cleaning, brushing teeth, etc.
This isn't essential, but useful for mild situations. Do not
use drinking water for these reasons if you're in a moderate
or extreme emergency.

Your water in your house is ultimately dependent on
electricity. While you may have had running water during
the last local blackout, a major blackout will shut down the
water processing and pumping stations. If you have a well,
the pump runs off electricity. Can you get water out of your
well without power?

Do you have pets? Add in water for them, but in
moderate or extreme emergencies, let them forage for
water. They can do it much better than you.

Quite a bit of the food you will have stored will require
water to prepare. That's why you might think the
recommended gallon a day seems high.

*We have water already stored in houses in places we
might not automatically think of:*
Our hot water heater contains a considerable amount.
There is a drain at the bottom. Make sure you have
something to collect the water in, open the drain, then open
a faucet to complete the water circuit. (Make sure, if not
already off, that you turn off the gas/power to the heater
before working on it. If the power/gas is already off and
comes on, make sure you immediately refill the heater
before turning it back on or else it can overheat.)

The water pipes in your house can be drained of the
water in them.

Our toilet tank (not the toilet bowl) contains fresh
water. Get over it and use it.

A swimming pool or hot tub contains non-potable water which you can make potable. These techniques are covered in Survival.

If you have adequate warning, you should fill every available container with potable water. Also fill all tubs and sinks.

Mod/Ex: Long term storage of a large supply of water:
Using milk containers or other thin plastic is not recommended for storing water as thin plastic degrades and will leak. You can use soda or juice bottles with thicker plastic. Glass is fine, except it is heavy and subject to breakage.

To re-use such containers, thoroughly clean them out with soap and water, then rinse completely, insuring there is no residual soap.

Sanitize these bottles by adding one teaspoon of un-scented chlorine bleach to every quart (note that bleach also has a shelf-life of six months, so make sure it is fresh). Shake the container, with the lid on, thoroughly sanitizing it. Empty, wash out with clean water. Then fill it and add two drops non-scented bleach and tightly seal the top.

Date the outside of the container with a permanent marker.

Store in a dry, cool place.

Rotate every six months.

If you're going with smaller sized containers like this, stagger filling them so that they all don't come due to be refilled at the same time which, according to Murphy's Law, is usually about the time you'll need the water. However, if necessary, consider this water potable in an emergency if it is your only option. The rotation is to err on the side of caution.

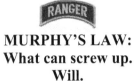

MURPHY'S LAW:
What can screw up.
Will.

There are larger size water containers for sale. There are fixed sided containers and collapsible bladders. If you want to store of large quantities of potable water, 55 gallon drums work well. Make sure they are food grade (HDPE #2).

Check stored water every two months and refill at a minimum of every six months. Remember, once you fill this barrel, you won't be able to move it because water is heavy. This is also something to factor in when considering how much water you can carry.

Water weighs 8.34 pounds per gallon. (3.78 Kg)

We'll cover this in more detail later, but you should carry water in your car. Store a case of water somewhere inside your vehicle for Mod/Ex. For Mild have two bottles within arm's reach of the driver's seat in case you are trapped.

Learn your local area (we'll cover this in detail in the Area Study). Do you have a natural source of drinkable water within walking distance? Is there one near your BOHS? Once more, you must consider any water in nature to be contaminated.

There are items that can be used to purify water and some of these will become part of your Grab-n-Go bags. These are:

Survival straw

Survival filter

Water purification tablets

Suggestions and links to these items are at the end of the book in the Appendix Gear.

Field expedient means for disinfecting water are covered under survival.

Task Nineteen
Mild: Water Checklist

Completed		Expiration date
	3 gallons of water per person 2 cases	Rotate every six months
	2 bottles of water in car.	Rotate every six months
	2 bottles of water in work/school GnG bag	Rotate every six months

Task Twenty Mod/Ex: Water Checklist

Completed		Expiration date
	Moderate: 3 gallons of water per person 2 cases	Rotate every six months
	Moderate: Portable water filter Katadyn Water Microfilter: https://amzn.to/2LBYcuE	Expiration date of cartridge
	Extreme: 30 gallons per person or more (10 cases, 55 gallon drum, etc)	Rotate every six months
	Mod/Ex: location of drinkable water source near home	Make sure it is safe
	Mod/Ex: GnG Bag: bottle of water purifying pills	Expiration date on bottle
	Mod/Ex GnG bag: Survival Straw LifeStraw Personal Water Filter: https://amzn.to/2V4uUJf	
	Mod/Ex: One case of water in car.	Rotate every six months
	Extreme: BOHS— drinkable water source near hide site.	Make sure it is safe

FOOD

Every time I go into the grocery store, I'm amazed at the amount and variety of food. Actually, I look like the guy at the end of *Hurt Locker*, staring at all the various types of cereal in utter confusion. When the checkout person asks me if I found everything, I tell them "No, and my wife will let me know when I get home."

Having gone without food for eight days during survival training and parachuted in with all the food (and ammunition and other gear) I was going to have for the next 30 days on an operation, I am very aware of the importance of food.

I'm also aware of how quickly the food in stores will go bad and rot within a few days with no power or being replaced. Most people have several days to a week's worth of food on hand in the refrigerator and pantry. If the power goes off, start on the food in the freezer first, then the refrigerator, as those will be good for only about three days.

In most situations after water, our next most urgent requirement is food. Actually, most people's minds turn to food before they think of water, even though the latter is more critical.

How much food do you have stored in your house?

What is the shelf life?

Emergency food should be outside the normal rotation of food you use daily, except as you need to rotate the stored food to keep from spoilage. This emergency food should be stored in a different location than your normal food supply. Keep track of expiration dates on a calendar.

As an aside, it can get complicated keeping track of various things you need to check on a regular basis. After years of trying different techniques, I've settled on coordinating all events on the same days and thus having a standard rotation schedule as follows:

Task Twenty-One
Mild: Rotation and Inspection Checklist

Rotate or Check Every:	Item
Month. (1st of each month)	Test fire alarms
Quarterly (1 Jan, 1 April, 1 July, 1 Oct)	Gas in spare cans, Power bars, emergency water in vehicle,
Semi-Annual (1 Jan, 1 July)	Replace fire alarm batteries; check first aid kits Conduct fire drill Check all emergency food
Annual (1 Jan)	Gng bags, check all
Every five years	Replenish emergency bars
Every ten years	Replace smoke alarms

The easiest way to decide what food to get is to store the non-perishable food you normally eat, keeping in mind expiration dates. This requires you to have a rotation plan. Do not put your rotation plan on your iCal or other electronic device. It must be a manual plan. In fact, back up all information you will need in a survival situation that is currently on an electronic platform on a manual platform. Such as this book. While reading this as an eBook is useful for preparation, you want a print copy for the actual emergency.

If you don't want to invest a lot of time into this, there are numerous companies that make and sell bulk packets of long-lasting food supplies (25 years in many cases). These sites even have survival food spreadsheets where you can calculate what you need. While this might not be the 'hard-core' survivalist way, it's a smart way. The upfront investment is worth the long-term comfort of mind. I have several of these buckets of food.

This is an important area. I believe you can do things the hard way or the easy way. Survival is hard. Preparing for it doesn't need to be. Experts have done much of the preparation for you; you just have to use them. However, I've also learned not to go cheap on certain life-saving items.

You must also factor in what it takes to prepare the food. For mild emergencies, you need food that doesn't require cooking.

Things to consider for food:

Shelf life?

How hard is it to prepare?

Weight to calorie ratio?

Percentages of macronutrients?

At this point you're tearing your hair out at the thought of doing all the research. You could, but here are basic suggestions:

Energy and protein bars. Any off the shelf brand will do for mild emergencies. If you want to fine tune things, go for ones that don't have too much salt and sugar, because those two ingredients will make you thirsty.

Task Twenty-Two Mild: Food Checklist

Completed		Expiration date
	3 days of non-perishable food. **2,400 calories per day per person**	Rotate as needed
	Non-electric can opener	
	Power Bars: **https://amzn.to/2Rd54DN**	Check Expiration date

Mod/Ex Food

Invest in emergency ration bars. They are a bit expensive, but you won't mind the outlay when you need them.

The ones I list all are 3600 calories, which in a survival situation equals 800 calories a day for three days. They contain a mixture of salt, carbohydrates, fat, protein and are usually enriched with daily requirements of minerals and vitamins. Some reasons to have these:

1.   They have a five year shelf life, so you can store them.

2.   They're compact (but heavy)

3.   They're ready to eat (no cooking)

4.   They can withstand wide temperature swings,

which helps with storage.

    5.   They don't make you thirsty.

I have ration bars in my vehicles, my Grab-n-Go bag, and in my cache at the GOHS. I recommend storing some at work. Even just one packet in each place makes a big difference; and it's less than two cups of extra-whatever-latte-frappe you order at Starbucks.

Some things to consider:

-Put them inside a large ziplock bag, because once you open the packet, the bars aren't individually sealed.

-They are emergency rations, not to be used if other rations are available.

-They are designed for survival not activity.

-They're heavy so many don't put them in Grab-n-Go bags, but I think the weight is worth it.

Mountain House Freeze Dried Meals. This is the same company that made the LRRP meals we loved in Special Operations. They don't take much water, but they do require cooking. Unless you're really hard core.

GORP or trail mix. This is a ready-made mixture, with a base of raisins and peanuts. There are many variations beyond that including items such as banana chips, oats, granola, etc. For high calorie situations such as winter warfare training, we added peanut M&Ms in the mixture.

Besides the food in your house, have a cache of food in a location away from your house. The reason for this is covered later under the Emergency Rally Point (ERP).

Task Twenty-Three. Mod/Ex: Food Checklist

Completed		Expiration date
	Moderate: A week's worth of non-perishable food. 2,400 calories per day per person	
	Extreme: A month's worth of non-perishable food. 2,400 calories per day per person Mountain House Essential Bucket: https://amzn.to/2BAkM21	
	Mod/Ex: Emergency Rations Grizzly Gear: https://amzn.to/2Lzqk1l ERbar: https://amzn.to/2SfllW4 DaTrex 3600: https://amzn.to/2LzqtBV	Check Expiration date
	Mod/Ex: A means of cooking food away from home. MSR Dragon Fly: https://amzn.to/2SgoTHz	Rotate as needed
	Mod/Ex: Scavenging, hunting and gathering. Covered under Survival.	
	Multivitamins: Two months worth	

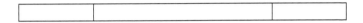

Mod/Ex: What kind of food?

There is, of course, more to food than just calories, and not all calories are created equal. You know this by the way you feel after eating different meals. Some give quick, readily accessible energy, while others make you feel slowed down and lethargic.

Most of us have a high intake of carbohydrates that give us a nonstop stream of energy. That intake flow is rarely interrupted for long periods of time.

Macronutrients are the keys to food and we focus essentially on carbohydrates, proteins and fats. Technically, water is one of these, but we've already covered that.

Getting more particular, the breakdown of our food should be:

Carbohydrates: 45% to 65% for everyone

Proteins: 10-35% for adults; 10 to 30% for children; 5-20% for infants

Fats: 20-35% for adults; 10-30% for children; 5-20% for infants

Specific caloric needs:

If you're one of those types, and you know who I'm talking about, and want to get into the specifics of how much food you need, here are some formulas the more mathematically inclined can play with, otherwise go with the 2,500 calories a day per person as a solid guideline with some buffer built in.

BMR is Basic Metabolic Rate. That's what the body consumes at rest in order to survive. BMR varies by height, weight, activity level and gender. Men tend to consume more calories than women on average.

Male BMR= 66 + (6.23 x weight in pounds) + (12.7 x height in inches) – (6.8 x age in years)

Female BMR= 655 + (4.35 x weight in pounds) + (4.7 x height in inches) – (6.8 x age in years)

Notice that the older you are, the less calories you need.

Then we can factor in you activity with the Harris Benedict Formula:

Sedentary: calories needed = BMR x 1.2

Lightly active: BMR x 1.375

Moderately active: BMR x 1.55

Very active: BMR x 1.725

Extra active (running from zombies active): BMR x 1.9

Extreme emergency food considerations:

I noted that a person can go several weeks without food. That, however, is stretching it. I've gone eight days without food; interestingly I stopped feeling hungry after a few days. However, the ability to function begins to degrade.

When our output exceeds our caloric intake these are the symptoms:

-physical weakness

-confusion, poor judgment, and disorientation

-weakened immune system

-inability to maintain body temperature which can lead to hypothermia, heat exhaustion/stroke

The Coast Guard has determined that with fresh water people can survive in a life raft 8 to 18 days without any food. The Coast Guard also believes you need a bare minimum of 800 calories a day for survival; but that's sitting in a life raft, not being very active and just focused on pure survival.

If you want to figure out exactly how much caloric intake you need, you can use the BMR formula above, then apply it to the projected emergency.

Hunting, gathering and scavenging food is covered later under Survival.

Food expiration dates:

There are some things to understand about this.

First, there are several terms stamped on the food. This is what they mean:

SELL BY: How long a store should display the product for sale. This is a guide for the store. It is optimum quality date, but food is still edible for a while after.

BEST IF USED BY OR BEFORE DATE: This is only about quality, not safety.

GUARANTEED FRESH DATE: This usually refers to bakery items. They will still be edible after that date.

USE BY DATE: This is the last recommended day to use the product at peak quality. It is still edible after this.

PACK DATE: This is on canned and packaged goods. This actually might not be clear as sometimes it's in code. It can be done by month-day-year as MMDDYY. Or it could be Julian calendar for the year by day, which means January is numbered 001-0031. December would be 334-365.

Foods not to eat past their expiration date?

Eggs. Deli meat. Mixed greens. Alfalfa sprouts. Oysters. Shrimp. Raw ground beef. Berries. Soft cheese. Chicken.

So how long is food usually good for?

Milk: a week after Sell By.

Eggs: Three to five weeks after you buy them. Double-grade A will go down a grade in a week, but are still edible.

Poultry and seafood: Cook or freeze within a day.

Beef and pork: Cook or freeze within three to four days.

Canned good: High acid foods such as tomato sauce can last to 18 months. Low acid such as canned green beans can last for five years. However, do not store these in a hot space. A dry, cool place, is best.

More on Food

While you already have an emergency food supply, here are some more considerations.

While you can get bulk supplies, in an extreme and extended emergency, a little variety is nice. While I do have bulk supplies of emergency food, I offset that with soups, noodles, and other long-lasting food stuffs. Many extreme survivalists go with staples such as wheat (do you have allergies, by the way, or any of your team?). We grow weary of eating the same food day after day. Even the Army mixes up their rations. Consider storing some spices. My team-members would carry various spices and sauces with them to "spice up" their bland rations in the field.

Stock up on vitamins, especially for children. Multi-vitamins work well and vitamin C is essential.

Consider 'goodies'. These are key for keeping up morale. While we can live on gruel for a long time, it's not fun living. While our mindset in an emergency is survival, as time goes on, there is a need to pick up spirits. While I was in 10th Special Forces we experimented with GORP (good old raisins and peanuts), aka trail mix. A mixture of peanuts, dried fruits such as bananas and raisins. We also tended to add in chocolate in the form of M&Ms. We carried a supply in our ruck and usually a ziplock bag in our outer shells for easy access while on the move. You can buy this already mixed at your local supermarket.

Be careful of your use of containers. Air locked containers are best to avoid spoilage. You do not want your food supply contaminated with water. Do not use trash can liners as they are sometimes treated with pesticides. In an earthquake zone don't store your food on high racks. They can topple and break the container.

Test and use your emergency food while replenishing. It's too late to learn how to cook and figure out how much you like your emergency food supply to do it during the emergency. Set aside time to try some of the meals. Learn how long it takes to cook. Also, use your emergency stove to cook. See how people react to the various items. Restock with these factors in mind.

But we're doing great. We've prepared for two of the five key areas!

FIRST AID

Triage priorities:
Breathing.
Bleeding.
Broken.

We check injured people in that order, so this give us our priority in terms of preparation.

It's the order in which a person dies. However, like everything else, there are exceptions. Arterial bleeding (spurting blood) can kill as quickly as lack of oxygen.

If injured, First Aid can quickly become the number one priority over food and water.

Spend money on well-stocked first aid kits. Also get at least one Quickclot bandage, a very effective way to stop bleeding. You will also need a first aid kit at your work, in your car, and in your Grab-n-Go bag and cached at your BOHS.

While it's better to actually do the first aid training, a mild baseline is to have the information at your fingertips.

The following Apps are free and the links are in the mild checklist further on.

First Aid (Red Cross):

The official American Red Cross First Aid app puts expert advice for everyday emergencies in your hand. With videos, interactive quizzes and simple step-by-step advice it's never been easier to know first aid. Features:

• Easy to use Spanish language toggle to switch translation directly inside the app.

• Simple step-by-step instructions guide you through everyday first aid scenarios.
• Fully integrated with 9-1-1 so you can call EMS from the app at any time.
• Videos and animations make learning first aid fun and easy.
• Preloaded content means you have instant access to all safety information at any time, even without reception or an Internet connection.

iTriage. iTriage is a free app that puts you at the center of your healthcare—anywhere, anytime. Search for health answers with iTriage Health, Doctor, Symptom & Healthcare Search app. Find medications, diseases, and medical locations.

CPR and Choking. Has video demonstration and audio instructions that you can quickly access. The first screen is two large buttons where you pick either CPR or Choking. Then you get the choice of adult/child/infant. Once you hit that, the video begins to play.

Medications
Medical supplies are going to be in great demand in an extreme emergency. You need at least a week's supply of whatever medications you take, preferably a month. If it appears that the extreme emergency will be of lasting duration, getting more of that medication is a priority along with learning what homeopathic substitutes are available in nature and how to prepare them.

Drug Expiration dates:
By law, an expiration date means the manufacturer guarantees full potency to at least 90% by that date, given proper storage. That doesn't mean the medication suddenly

goes bad. Companies are not required by law to test beyond that date for potency.

Drugs that should never be used past their expiration date:

Anticonvulsants - narrow therapeutic index
Dilantin, phenobarbital - very quickly lose potency
Nitroglycerin - very quickly lose potency
Warfarin - narrow therapeutic index
Procan SR - sustained release procainamide
Theophylline - very quickly lose potency
Digoxin - narrow therapeutic index
Thyroid preparations
Paraldehyde
Oral contraceptives
Epinephrine - very quickly lose potency
Insulin - very quickly lose potency
Eye drops - eyes are particularly sensitive to any bacteria that might grow in a solution once a preservative degrades.

The reality is a drug starts to lose potency from the moment it's manufactured. However, it doesn't suddenly go bad at the expiration date. Even though your meds might have passed the expiration date, they can still be useful in an emergency situation. Research indicates that most drugs, properly stored, retain 90% of their effectiveness for at least five years after the expiration date, sometimes longer.

The most stable are tablets and capsules. Those that are in a solution or a reconstituted suspension do not last as long. The Department of Defense actually studied this under a program called the Shelf Life Extension Program (SLEP). It found that 88% of 122 different drugs stored under ideal conditions should have their expiration dates extended more than 1 year, with an average extension of 66 months, and a maximum extension of 278 months.

Even more astounding was research where eight medications that had expired 28 to 40 years ago were tested. Their 15 active ingredients were: aspirin, amphetamine, phenacetin, methaqualone, codeine, butalbital, caffeine, phenobarbital, meprobamate, pentobarbital, secobarbital, hydrocodone, chlorpheniramine, and acetaminophen. Eleven of the fourteen drug compounds were always present in concentrations of at least 90% of the amount indicated on the drug label, which is generally recognized as the minimum acceptable potency.

The only report I could find of human toxicity from an expired drug was tetracycline. Be aware that this is not a well-researched field as it isn't in the pharmaceutical companies interest. I am NOT recommending you take expired meds. I am saying it makes sense to properly and securely store expired meds and use only as a last resort.

Drugs in liquid form are not as stable. Drugs requiring the addition of a solvent before taking or administering aren't as stable. They are also susceptible to freezing.

In the case of liquids for things like contacts or eye drops, the danger is microbial growth. Injectable drug that have become cloudy or discolored should not be used.

Mod/Ex keys to first aid:

Train, train, train. CPR, stopping bleeding, stabilizing broken limbs. All are priorities. Learn how to recognize and deal with hypothermia, heat exhaustion and dehydration.

Stay up to date on physical exams.

A critical part of first aid that many people ignore in survival situations is personal hygiene. Preventing illness is more important than treating it.

Prepare, prepare, prepare. Antibiotics are critical. So are bandages. Splints. Medicine.

As part of your Area Study (coming soon) you will be familiar with health threats in your locale. Be prepared for them. This includes not just flora and fauna threats, but environmental ones.

If you wear glasses, have a backup pair. Even using old prescription glasses is better than nothing. Don't throw those glasses away, store them. If you wear contacts, make sure you have a back-up pair of glasses.

Those who need them should have medical alert badges on at all times.

Stop putting off your physical and your dental exam. You'll really regret it if you ever are in a situation where you can't get one. Get dental work done as soon as possible or else envision Tom Hanks with an ice skate working on you.

When building your team, a person with medical training should be a high priority.

Every member of your team should receive basic first aid training. This goes beyond the local CPR course. The chances that you will have to perform CPR are higher in day-to-day living then in a survival situation, as other types of injuries will be more prevalent. A few hours spent going over first aid basics can yield great results.

The Red Cross offers on line First Aid courses you can take at your own pace.

Red Cross on line First Aid Courses:
http://www.redcross.org/take-a-class/first-aid/first-aid-training/first-aid-online

More on how to actually do First Aid in *Survival*. A great help to being able to conduct first aid, though, is to have the proper supplies in place beforehand.

Task Twenty-Four. Mild: First Aid Checklist

First Aid kit: Adventure Med Kit Weekender: http://amzn.to/2f3gh4c		
Quikclot sponge: http://amzn.to/2fkHgMr		
Red Cross First Aid App (Apple): https://itunes.apple.com/us/app/first-aid-by-american-red/id529160691?mt=8 **(Android):** https://play.google.com/store/apps/details?id=com.cube.arc.fa&hl=en		
iTriage App (Apple): https://itunes.apple.com/us/app/itriage-symptom-checker/id304696939 **(Android):** https://play.google.com/store/apps/details?id=com.healthagen.iTriage		
CPR and choking app: (Apple): https://itunes.apple.com/app/cpr-choking/id314907949 **CPR and Choking (Android):** https://play.google.com/store/apps/details?id=org.learncpr.videoapp		
Medical Alert Badges as needed		
Annual Physical		
Glasses as backup if use contacts--Extra pair of glasses		
1 week supply of medications		
Car: First Aid kit: Adventure Med Kit Weekender: http://amzn.to/2f3gh4c		

Task Twenty-Five
Mod/Ex: First Aid Checklist

First Aid Kit: **Lifeline 4038 Hard Shell:** http://amzn.to/2eSbS3H		
Trauma Pack w/ Quik-Clot https://amzn.to/2Rbyxy0		
Universal Splint, rolled: http://amzn.to/2f3eCfe		
Recon Tourniquet: https://amzn.to/2Lzt1jt		
Complete a CPR course		
Complete a First Aid Course		
1 month of medications; know homeopathic replacements		
GnG bag: First Aid kit: Adventure Med Kit Weekender: http://amzn.to/2f3gh4c		

SHELTER

Think of the actual word: Shelter. The dictionary defines it as "*a place giving temporary protection from bad weather or danger.*" It protects us from cold, the sun, wind, rain and snow. While shelter is normally third or fourth on the list of priorities, in extreme environments or weather, it can easily become the number one priority, because, as the Rule of Threes notes: we can survive only 3 hours with an unregulated body temperature.

Optimally our home will be our shelter. The keys I list below will apply largely to that. I'm not going to list things that would normally be in a home such as blankets, pots, pans, etc.

Do not underestimate the importance of shelter to morale. Lack of shelter can lead to fatigue and exhaustion. It can also make a person feel lost and anchor-less. People without shelter can quickly gain the thousand-yard-stare of passive helplessness and lose the will to survive.

Clothing:
Normally we don't think of our clothes as shelter, but they are the most important aspect of protecting ourselves from the environment. We have to make the shift from thinking of clothes in terms of fashion, to that of functionality and protection.

What do you normally wear? How effective would it be in an emergency? Would you be able to walk a mile in adverse weather in the clothes and footwear you normally wear to work/school or traveling?

Footwear and socks:
A priority is to make sure you have a good pair of broken in walking shoes/boots at work/school and in your car. Some years ago, during a bad ice storm in Atlanta, many people tried walking home from work, or their

abandoned car, in the shoes they wear at work and direly wished they had been better prepared. Ever since learning of this, I've had a pair of broken in boots along with several pairs of socks stuffed in them, in my Jeep.

Having served in the Infantry and then Special Forces, the importance of proper footwear cannot be over-emphasized. At the very least have some kind of workout shoes that you've broken in. Optimally, you would want something, that provides some ankle support and a degree of waterproofing. Footwear is so much a matter of personal opinion, the main thing to consider is how far can you walk in it?

While running and hiking shoes are popular, I'm a fan of boots for survival. For warm and moderate climates, I use the old standby of Army jungle boots. For colder environments I have a pair of Gore-Tex boots. For extreme cold, you might consider vapor boots or Micky Mouse boots as we called them in the army. These are large, rubber boots with air pumped into them. The air acts as insulation. They are warm, but you will sweat profusely in them, so make sure you have plenty of socks. Remember, as clothing and socks get dirty, even though you might dry them out, they are not as effective.

Whatever parts of your boot are leather should be treated to make them waterproof and soft. I use mink oil. Actually, I use mink oil on any leather product I have. Rubbing it in will eventually make the leather water resistant and more supple.

Break your boots in. An emergency is not the first time to put your boots on and start walking.

For most environments, in conjunction with long pants and boots, I use boot bands. These are stretchable bands. You roll the bottom of you pant leg inward with the boot band inside. This fixes the pants to the boots. This will prevent little critters like ticks from getting up inside your pants.

Do not go cheap on footwear.

Remember, that between you and the footwear is another key piece of shelter: socks. Of all articles of clothing to consider putting in my rucksack for a deployment, the priority was an adequate number of socks. Your socks need to be dry, so your feet stay dry, thus a change is critical. And even dry socks, if they are dirty, are less effective. There are socks with different materials specifically designed for working out or hiking.

An army travels on its feet. This lesson was drummed into me from my first day on the Plain at West Point. Any Infantry officer can tell you that taking care of his soldier's feet is one of the key components of his job. Your body travels on its feet. A breakdown there, and you're stuck. If you have not experienced an open blister, you have no idea how quickly such an apparently minor injury can stop you.

Layering.

The primary rule of outdoor survival is to STAY DRY. Hypothermia is the #1 killer of people outdoors. It can happen very quickly, particularly if you get wet. I've seen highly trained soldiers succumb to this, especially if you combine this with being dehydrated.

Your clothing should keep you warm and also provide insulation when wet. For this reason, avoid cotton, since it loses all its insulating properties when wet. Remember this saying: 'Cotton is rotten.' This particularly applies when considering your underwear and t-shirts. Most jeans are made of cotton and are not a good choice despite their durability and cowboys.

Wool is a much better choice, maintaining up to 80% of its warmth even when wet, although it is slow to dry. There are many fabrics that provide warmth, even when wet, and also dry quickly. A key is to keep your clothing from getting wet in the first place with an outer, water-proof layer.

How well would your clothing stand up to an emergency environment? The best way to shop for good emergency clothing is to go your local camping store and see what they sell to people who spend a lot of time outdoors in the local area.

The key to clothing is layering. You start with what's closest to your body. Even if you're not going to be in a cold environment, layering is still a key concept to understand. It is important to not only keep warm, but dry, no matter where you are. Often, in the desert, while the day might be hot, the night can easily drop below freezing, depending on the time of year.

Layering works in threes:

Inner layer. Whatever is directly against your skin. The goal is to wick moisture away from your skin to the next layer. Your body heat does the work, so the better the material for this, the less energy your body has to expend. This layer should have a snug fit around your body, as the body's heat is what wicks the moisture. The material used should absorb less than one percent of moisture. In very cold environments, you want to have hoods, glove liners, and neck wraps.

Middle layer. This layer is your insulation. Its primary purpose is to keep you warm, while it also helps wick away the moisture to the outer layer. This middle layer must move the moisture outward while keeping heat in. When you think middle layer, consider several garments instead of just one, so you can adjust layers as the temperature changes or your level of exertion changes. One thing you want to prevent at all costs in cold weather is sweating inside your layers.

Outer layer. While the first two layers are focused on keeping warmth in and wicking moisture away, the primary purpose of the outer layer is to battle outside elements, primarily wind and moisture. It should also have the ability to wick away moisture from inside. If this layer only repels rain and wind, it's called a shell. Usually, though, this outer layer will have an insert that can be added or removed as needed. It should be breathable to allow moisture to wick out. Gore-Tex is a commonly used outer material. If your outer layer is not breathable, be careful of building up perspiration on the interior.

Keep in mind that sweating in a cold weather environment can be a killer as you are covering your body with moisture. When we were at 14,000 feet altitude, in eight feet of snow, and getting ready to move out on our skies, with our large rucksacks, I gave time warnings, starting at five minutes from move out. The purpose of this was to give my men time to strip down. As we got closer to moving, we'd take off our outer layer, storing it in the ruck. Then just before move out, we'd take off our middle layers. It was very cold and uncomfortable to do this, but a few minutes after tossing our rucks on our backs and moving out on skis, we were working up a lot of heat. If we were still wearing those other layers, we'd be sweating profusely. The moment we stopped, that sweat would either freeze or be trapped against our body.

Most of your body heat is lost through your head.

A watch cap is indispensable in a cold environment. I carry a couple, to allow me to dry the unused one out next to my body. I view those the same as socks.

For hot and/or jungle/desert environments, I wear a billed cap or, better, a bush hat. I prefer to wear long sleeves and pants in hot weather, instead of shorts and short-sleeve shirts. This is for protection from the sun and the environment. A light material, with a light color.

Remember, black absorbs the sun's rays. There are pants and shirts now where the lower leg and arm parts can be removed so you can have the best of both worlds.

Home:

Our home is our primary shelter. Given you've already covered the prior areas, it should be well stocked with food and water and a first aid kit.

When I watch reality shows about survival on TV, the people who have built their homes into bunkers and stored up a year's worth of supplies make me shake my head. First, the fact they're advertising this on TV is, well, dumb. But the other factor is this: if I were the truly lazy survivalist, and a sociopath, I would target known survivalists in my area, let them do all the preparation work, then ambush them and take their house and supplies. I have no doubt this will occur in extreme emergencies. Desperate people are dangerous people. In fact, one of the largest flaws I see in many survival guides is the focus on preparing a static survival base, which, in extreme emergencies, is simply building an attractive target. This is why you're learning to be flexible in this book in order to face an array of levels of emergencies.

Task Twenty-Six
Mild: Shelter Checklist

	Walking boots/shoes at work/school/car with socks	
	Proper clothing for your environment	
	Gloves, hat	
	Car: rain jacket or poncho	
	Car: Blanket	

Mod/Ex: Shelter

There are items that will go in your Grab-n-Go bags for shelter. These are a tent or at the very least a poncho. An emergency sleeping bag. Extra clothing. Hat. Gloves. Etc. All of these are listed in that section.

With all shelter, including clothing, consider two extremes. First, that you want to be seen by rescuers. The second option is that you don't want to be seen by others. This would probably be the norm in an extended, extreme emergency, where law and order has broken down.

Your gear should naturally lean toward the second choice (not being seen), while you have specific equipment—signal panel, signal mirror, strobe light, etc.—that allows you to signal rescuers. Thus your bag for Grab-n-Go, your clothing, your tent, etc. should be subdued or camouflage colored for your environment. While my Jeep is orange (bought it used that way), I carry subdued plasti-dip pain in case of extreme emergency and I need to camouflage it.

Task Twenty-Seven. Mod/Ex Shelter Checklist

	Walking boots/shoes at work/school/car with socks	
	Proper outdoor clothing for your environment	
	Watch cap and/or boonie hat: Watch cap: https://amzn.to/2LvL5uX Boonie Hat: https://amzn.to/2QKgI9X	
	Car: rain jacket or poncho Rain jacket: Poncho: https://amzn.to/2LvsWx8	
	Car: Blanket and Emergency Bivy sack: https://amzn.to/2R7FLmP	
	GnG: As per the environment, check GnG section.	

FIRE

Fire can be our friend or our enemy, so let's cover it both ways.

In our normal civilized world, fire is considered a luxury for those who have a fireplace in their house, but you have to realize that fire actually affects a lot of your day-to-day life. Fire is usually how our home is heated and a lot of our food prepared. In our house, in a mild to moderate emergency, there is a chance we will need fire, whether it is to purify water, cook food or to keep warm.

The immediate keys to fire preparation:

Do you have a way to cook food if your gas/power is turned off? Without the microwave or stove, how will you prepare a meal? You can invest in a small camping stove with disposable tanks for not much money. But consider how much fuel you will need proportionate to the emergency food supply you have. Test cook meals until you use up one tank.

Do you have a way to provide or conserve warmth in your house if your power/gas is turned off? This does not necessarily have to be a fire. Blankets and clothing can make do in most cases.

Do you have a fireplace in your house? If its wood burning, how much wood do you have on hand? Have you stored it so that it's dry? Do you have kindling or fire starter?

Is your fireplace gas? Can it be converted to wood? If it is gas or propane, can you start it with the power off without blowing up the house? Check the owner's manual.

Does your propane heat work even if the power is off? Do you know how to manually start it?

Do you have an outdoor means of fire? A barbecue? Fire pit? Make sure you have enough fuel for this fire.

Do you have a way to start a fire? I carry a half dozen lighters with me in the field, along with field expedient fire-starters.

Consider that fire is a beacon, both through light at night and smoke in the day and smell around the clock. This can be useful in a rescue situation. In an extreme survival situation, be aware you might be signaling to the wrong people.

In the Grab-n-Go bag section, I discuss the various fire starters you should have.

How to start a field expedient fire is discussed under Survival.

Fire, however, can also be our enemy. The following statistics are surprising to most people. They were to me when I researched them.

RANGER	
FIRE	
Number of home first your household can expect in an average lifetime.	5
Chances your household will have a reported home fire in an average lifetime.	1 in 4
Chances someone in your household will suffer a fire injury in an average lifetime	1 in 10
Chances someone in your household will suffer a reported injury in a fire in an average lifetime.	1 in 89

Fire Prevention

You not only have to be prepared to start a fire, but you need to be prepared to put out a fire.

You need a fire extinguisher in your kitchen. It should be a chemical-based extinguisher, not a water-based one. In the event of a grease or electrical fire, a water-based on causes more problems by spreading the flames.

It's also recommended you have an extinguisher for every floor of your house. Make sure everyone knows where they are and how to use them. You should also carry a fire extinguisher in your car.

In a typical home fire, you often only have a few minutes to escape. Since smoke can be contained by doors and levels, you must have several alarms throughout your house. It is recommended that you have:

A minimum of one smoke alarm per floor.

A smoke alarm in every bedroom.

A smoke alarm outside every sleeping area.

The type recommended are a mixture of ionization and photoelectric alarms. Ionization may detect invisible particles associated with fast burning fires while photoelectric detect visible particles associated with moldering fires.

Alarms are either battery powered or hard-wired into the house. In the case of the latter, it should have a battery backup in case the power goes out.

A CO_2 alarm is recommended for every floor. Remember that CO_2 is present with all fires, but also can be present without a fire.

Heat alarms are useful, especially in the kitchen since there might often be smoke from cooking that will cause a smoke alarm to go off. However, they are not a substitute for smoke alarms as they do not react to smoke. Heat alarms are useful in attics, furnace rooms and garages.

Test all alarms monthly. Pick a specific day, perhaps the first Saturday of every month, and test. Replace batteries every six months, regardless of whether its indicated or not. All alarms should be replaced every ten years.

Take a look out of all your windows. Can you get out and to the ground safely? My wife looked out the master bedroom in one house we were renting and while it was on the main floor from the front, it was three stories up from the rear. We bought an emergency three-story ladder that you can throw out the window.

How to react in a fire is covered in Survival.

Task Twenty-Eight
Mild: Fire Checklist

	Fire extinguisher in kitchen	
	Fire extinguisher in each floor and near fireplaces	Check Every 6 months
	Fire extinguisher in car	Check Every 6 months
	Study fire drill safety in Survival portion and share with household	Check Every 6 months
	Fire drill in household every six months	
	Designate IRP in case of fire	
	Emergency ladder in all bedrooms above the first floor sufficient to reach the ground from a window. First Alert 2-Story Escape Ladder: https://amzn.to/2V65M4Z First Alert 3-Story Escape Ladder: https://amzn.to/2SdhatX	

Task Twenty-Nine
Mod/Ex : Fire Checklist

	A means of cooking meals in home if power is out.	
	Storm proof lighters (least 1 each home, GnG, car) **Storm proof lighters:** https://amzn.to/2Cv8yt7	
	Storm proof matches (1 ea GnG, home): https://amzn.to/2V5tEWe	
	Portable Stove (same as Food, Mod/Ex) **MSR Dragon Fly:** https://amzn.to/2SgoTHz	
	Extreme: Learn how to start a fire with items found in nature	

The Places for Which to Plan

The basic places to plan for are home, work/school and car/traveling. We've covered most of the home information already. We're adding some additional information for that and then specific information about the other locations.

HOME

Now that you've completed your Area Study, you need to prepare your home in the order of the probability of events that could occur based on that and also the likelihood of emergencies.

You've already prepared your water and food to at least the mild level. That's puts you far ahead of everyone else.

Stay informed about current and pending conditions. In some cases, such as hurricanes, you will have days of warning. Everyone in your survival team should contact each other the second anyone hears about a potential emergency in your area using the alert system you filled out at the beginning of this book.

Find out if your community has a disaster plan and warning systems.

Make sure everyone knows the IRP and ERP.

Make sure your out of town contact is up to speed on your plans. If you have to evacuate, they're ready for you to show up?

Make sure your insurance is up to date.

Earlier I described all the water sources in your house. If you have time, stock up on water in every possible holder, including bathtubs.

Have a physical calendar in your house, perhaps on the fridge, but somewhere you can see it every day. On it list the things that need to be checked on a routine basis. Cross them off as they get checked. Do not count on an electronic calendar.

Have all your key documents and records in a fireproof, secure place, that is mobile. There are small lockboxes that do this. The items to put in it are below. Also scan all key documents and store them in the cloud. It's worthwhile to go through your house and video everything in it and then store that recording in several places in case you need to make a claim. When you do this video, make sure all your drawers and doors are open so contents can be seen. Store the video somewhere outside of the house. Digitize it and put it in the cloud and also on thumb drives.

Task Thirty. Mild: Scan and store in cloud and on thumb drive the following documents. Then put in a mobile, fireproof secure box

Stored	Scanned	Cloud	Documents
			Birth Certificates
			Passports/Visas
			Home insurance documents
			Car insurance documents and registration
			Health insurance documents/Medical Cards
			Employment records
			Tax returns
			Drivers licenses
			Social Security Card
			Back-up ID (student ID, military, VA, etc.)
			Credit Cards
			Medical history
			Power of attorney
			Wills
			Concealed carry license
			Important phone numbers
			Titles/Deeds/etc
			Marriage License
			Financial accounts with account #, phone #, address,
			All military and VA records
			Thumb drive with video of house and all contents

Mild: Home Safety: Gas, Propane and Water
During many emergencies that threaten your home, it is wise to shut off your gas/propane. This greatly reduces the chance of fire, especially following earthquakes, tornadoes, hurricanes and floods.

To shut off the natural gas, turn the valve one-quarter (90 degrees) in either direction, if it's a valve. Have you checked your shut off? Does it turn? Often they might have become lodged in place. Make sure it turns and keep a wrench nearby just in case.

To shut off propane, turn the valve on the tank to the right all the way until it stops. For almost all valves and screws remember the says righty-tighty/lefty-loosey.

If you smell rotten eggs or hear hissing, shut off the gas.

If you have a buried propane tank, know where it is and where the lines run.

To shut off water at the house, find the main valve into the house. This could be key to keeping what water there is in the house, in it. If water mains break, and you're still connected to the water system, water will drain out of your house. Make sure you know where this shut off in the house is. While you might shut off the water by the meter, this is much more difficult and requires tools. Do you know where your water meter is?

EVACUATION
If you have to evacuate, pre-planning can save time and grief.

First, everything can be replaced except people! In extreme emergencies get out NOW and forget about taking anything. Wildfires, tsunamis and other events occur so quickly that seconds count. Get out!

If you are certain you have some time, having a checklist that you develop listing items to be taken in order of priority and where they are located will save confusion and time. I guarantee that without a checklist I'd forget half the things I need since I can have a thought, go up the stairs and forget what the thought is by the time I get to the top. I call this document my Bug Out list and have it on my phone and also printed in the top drawer of my desk. It lists the places in the house, garage, and vehicles where items are and then specifies the items. This allows me, for example, to go to the basement and grab everything I need from there on one trip. I even have to list where everything is in my Jeep because I have a lot of stuff in there and forget where, for example, I put the lugnut lock adapter, which is rather important when I have a flat.

Since this is personal, I recommend making your own form and filling it out. Some items that should be on it:

Lock box from above; GnG bags; medications; weapons; ammunition; spare gas cans; cell phone charge; computer and plug; home first aid kit; key tools; extra outdoor clothing (specified, such as gloves, hats, etc) and on and on. Once you've gone through all the Task Checklists in preparing you'll have a good idea of what you need.

Defense and the Safe Room

If you consider your home is your castle, then think about what the term castle means. It's a place of safety. Of defense.

Let me state up front I believe that the best defense is to not to have to defend yourself. Hiding works well. Retreating is also a good option.

We don't discuss weapons or using them much in this manual because there are two basic rules to firearms:

1. If I pull a firearm on someone, I must be prepared to use it.
2. If I use it, it is for lethal purposes.

Pulling a firearm escalates any situation into life or death. An extreme emergency. Avoid this at ALL cost.

When you use the term 'safe room' remember that it means two different things. FEMA looks at a safe room as a place where you can survive extreme weather. Security experts view a safe room as a place where you can outlast a home invasion. One is natural, the other man-made.

Mod/Ex Safe Room

FEMA safe room guidelines web site:
https://www.fema.gov/residential-safe-rooms

I won't go into it this in detail because you can go to the source document. Also, it requires engineering most likely beyond the capabilities of most do-it-yourselfers.

Your "safe room" can vary depending on the threat. Under hurricanes and tornadoes in Survival, I list where the best places to go are.

To guard against home invasion, consider this: the more you secure your house from someone getting in, the more you imprison yourself. If the fear of looters and criminals is so great during an emergency, retreat to your ERP, link up with your team and wait it out.

Have you looked at your home in terms of defensibility? If you don't have a military background, this might be a difficult thing to accomplish. Do you understand fields of fire, obstacles, cover, concealment? Again, discretion is the better part of valor.

I've looked at safe rooms in houses and to me, they look like prisons, unless it was a natural disaster such as a tornado. An issue to consider even for weather safe rooms: what if everything collapses down around you? How will you get out? Will rescuers know you are in that room? I think a weather safe room is a good idea, but think past the weather to rescue. Do you have a plan? In a way, if you think it through, you're caught in a Catch-22 here: if people know about your safe room in order to rescue you, then people know about your safe room. If you follow.

Again, as I keep pointing out in this book, one size does not fit all. For me, I prefer freedom of movement. But if I lived in a tornado zone, I would definitely have a weather safe room. Having lived in a hurricane zone, evacuation is the option to be taken over a safe room.

There are other reasons for safe rooms: terrorist attacks, especially with biological or chemical weapons.

Here are some guidelines for safe rooms:

A room with no windows.

Preferably a room with running water and a toilet. Or else you will need a chemical toilet. Remember the water and electricity can be cut off externally.

A landline phone.

Have heavy plastic and duct tape handy to seal any cracks if need be.

Since it's the most secure place in your house, this should be where your valuables are stored.

Don't call it a 'panic room' as that could make people panic.

Consider it a point of retreat until the threat goes away or help comes.

Do not leave the safe room until the threat is gone.

When you go to your safe room, take your GnG bag with you.

WORK/SCHOOL

The key to preparedness at work/school is to have your work/school Grab-n-Go bag on hand which is covered in the next chapter.

In an emergency your priority is to stay safe. Then to link up with your A-Team either at home, the IRP, or the ERP. A critical factor is who goes where and that has to be decided beforehand.

Sit down with your A-Team and discuss the possibilities of what happens if there is an emergency and cell phones don't work, yet everyone is in different places. What are the variables? How will you meet? Will you have time limits?

For example:

We meet at the home as long as it is viable given the emergency. If the home is abandoned, a note will be left in a waterproof container (an empty, closed water bottle will do) at the IRP, indicating whether the next step is the ERP or some other location. Always consider time limits.

It is instinctual for parents to head toward the school to get their children during an emergency. Do you know what the school's emergency plans are? Do you have the contact number for the school in order to be able to check? For the school district? Do your children know what to do if they have to leave the school? If you go to pick them up while they are coming home and you miss each other, do they know what to do if you aren't there?

Think of various scenarios and how your A-Team would deal with them if your cell phones don't work.

What are your work place's emergency plans? Most likely they have some, but they might be limited to evacuating the building.

What if you're trapped there?

Besides your own personal Grab-n-Go bag, your work place should have (your school should too, but that's usually at the discretion of the powers-that-be):

Task Thirty-One. Mild: Emergency equipment checklist for work/school

Completed	Item
	Battery operated emergency radio and/or TV
	Non-perishable 3 day supply of food for each person
	Bottled water for 3 days for each employee (2 cases per)
	Blankets, pillows, cots
	First aid kits
	First aid manual
	Flashlights, batteries, light sticks
	Toolkit
	Whistle, flare, to signal for help
	VS-17 or similar panel to signal for help, especially if forced to roof
	A designated IRP for all personnel outside the building
	Tarps, heavy duty plastic trash bags and duct tape
	Everyone knows building evacuation routes
	Emergency drills at least every six months/as required by law

Are there special considerations for your workplace and what its business is?

If you work in a very tall building do you know your options for getting out? Your escape route via stairwells down (never use the elevator)? Can you get to the roof if need be? Remember that helicopters might have problems getting close to the building if there is a fire. There are companies that are now making extended range escape possible using escape chutes and long range abseils (rappels). Consider even the possibility of base jumping. It might sound outrageous, but the lowest base jump ever recorded was only a little over 100 feet, which is roughly 10 stories. Many people work on a floor higher than 10 feet.

The most important thing for work is to have your work Grab-n-Go bag ready.

CAR/TRAVELING

Most people spend a considerable amount of time in their car, whether it's a road trip or a daily commute. What can you do to prepare and make traveling safer?

If your car doesn't have automatic running lights, turn on parking lights and leave them on while driving. Do it automatically. I turn on my Jeep fog and parking lights as soon as I turn on the ignition.

Buy good tires. Replace them before they reach safety limits. Replace all of them at the same time (my wife reminds me of this often for some reason). Rotate tires as instructed if you have a full size spare. Make sure your tire pressure is correct. Tires keep you on the road. Which I have found useful.

Don't let your gas level fall below half a tank. Yes, I know some of you are daredevils. You want to see how far you can go with the needle at empty, like Kramer in *Seinfeld*. Don't. In the Army, when I was in mechanized Infantry, it was a court martial offense if one of your armored vehicles ran out of fuel. Get in the habit of every time your gauge hits half, to top off. Do it for a month and it will be instinctual. And your significant other will never yell at you again for running out of gas. And you'll be damn happy to have that fuel as others wait in line after the hurricane.

If there is water on the road ahead and you don't know how deep it is, DO NOT attempt to drive through. At Fort Hood, Texas, the road would dip down into a dry gulch and there would be markers on the side of the culvert indicating the high point during flash flooding. It was often well over the roof of the car. Last year several soldiers died trying to cross one of those roads.

Hydroplaning: Did it, done it, won't ever drive fast on wet roads again. Roads are most dangerous just as it starts to rain as oil and other liquids already deposited on it rise. But in heavy rain, the road could be covered by more water than can be drained. Hydroplaning occurs when there is more water on the road than your tires can push away. The tires are then literally lifted on a sheet of water, losing your traction.

Unlike in the *Walking Dead*, gas has a shelf life. It begins to break down and is worthless after roughly three to six months. Gas with higher levels of ethanol breaks down more quickly.

You can add STA-BIL fuel stabilizer to gas you store or to gas power equipment you don't use often. The manufacturer claims it will keep gas usable up to two years. I think a year is pushing it. I rotate the gas in my emergency supplies quarterly and add Sta-Bil each time.

Carrying a battery powered siphon device is a smart move, as well as saving you inhaling gas through a hose.

RANGER	
I use Rotopax to carry extra gas, water and supplies. Their flat shape makes them easier to place on or inside your vehicles.	
Rotopax 2 gallon water can	https://amzn.to/2rYyHL5
Rotopax 2 gallon equipment holder	https://amzn.to/2BJTczn
FuelPax 4.5 gallon gas can	https://amzn.to/2AgWGt9
Rotopax 3.5 gallon gas can	https://amzn.to/2V9Iifn

Diesel lasts longer than gas, six months to a year.

An emergency 12 volt jump starter is an extremely useful device. Not only will it start your car if your battery is dead, it also is a power supply you can use in a pinch for your cell phone.

Have a little hammer/cutter device that allows you to smash open your window and cut loose from your seat belt in case the car goes into the water. Place this device within easy arms reach of your seat. There are also spring loaded car window breakers. They're called LifeHammers.

Besides your car Grab-nGo bag, here are some items you should have in your vehicle:

(It might be easier for many of these items to purchase a pre-packaged roadside emergency kit such as first listed).

Task Thirty-Two
Mild: Car equipment checklist

	Pre-packaged Roadside emergency kit (shown below and check the site to see what it holds) https://amzn.to/2CylcaV **This contains some of the items below—full list follows.**
	2 bottles of water
	Fire extinguisher: https://amzn.to/2V4u8fz
	Driver's license, proof of insurance, insurance company contact number
	Cell phone charger cable
	First Aid kit: Adventure Med Kit Weekender: http://amzn.to/2f3gh4c
	Reflective warning triangles: https://amzn.to/2SknVKE
	Flashlight with red warning flasher
	Blanket and Emergency bivy sack: https://amzn.to/2R7FLmP
	Life Hammer: https://amzn.to/2A8HL4r
	Ice scraper
	Work gloves
	Flat tire inflation canister: https://amzn.to/2CvN7s6
	Road maps as already designated under GPS/Maps
	Walking shoes/boots and socks as already designated
	Keychain pill fob with extra medication: https://amzn.to/2V9spoX

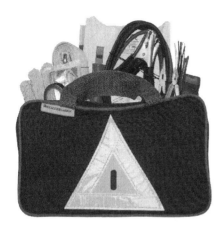

Roadside Emergency Kit
Includes - First Aid Kit,
Jumper Cables, Tow Rope, and
many other Supplies - 106
Pieces for assistance with
most Roadside Emergencies

Task Thirty-Three
Mod/Ex: Car equipment checklist

	Case of water or the equivalent (minimum 3 gallons)
	Collapsible Snow Shovel (based on Area Study) https://amzn.to/2rWOKc9
	Toolkit
	Jumper cables
	GoTreads Emergency Traction: https://amzn.to/2ShCnCV
	Tow straps
	Poncho: https://amzn.to/2LvsWx8
	Road side flares (I prefer battery power lights): https://amzn.to/2CF8nvt
	Spare fuses for your vehicle
	Spare bulbs for turn signals and brake lights for your vehicle
	Extra quart of oil
	Duct tape
	Battery powered siphon: https://amzn.to/2SegtAI
	Multipurpose tool: https://amzn.to/2Lzt3bh **and/or** **Leatherman Crunch tool:** https://amzn.to/2BD3lxR
	Emergency Battery Charger: https://amzn.to/2LwEu3p
	Survival radio: https://amzn.to/2BBBaiN

Do you know where your spare tire is? How to change it? Is it standard size or only a temporary spare good for emergency use? If that's the case, then don't drive as if you have regular tires and realize it's good for perhaps fifty miles. Some cars have tire mobility kits instead of spares; this consists of an inflator and sealant.

Travel

When you are traveling, there are specifics for air, rail, ferry, sea travel that are covered later in this book in Survival. A key thing is to do a quick area study of where you are going. What are the possible emergencies and threats?

Are you going to an area with a more primitive standard of living? Do you need water purification tablets? First aid kit? Here are some items to carry with you while traveling.

Task Thirty-Four. Mild: Travel checklist

	Passport and copy of your passport. Scan your passport and upload it to the cloud
	Health insurance card
	Extra credit card carried separate from your wallet/purse along with copy of passport
	Written list of emergency contact numbers (in case you lose your cell phone)
	Prepaid long distance calling card
	A few blank checks if you don't normally carry your check book

	Medication plus at least 3 extra days than the trip is planned
	Protein bars
	Cash

The Grab-n-Go Bag

Now that you know the five key elements of survival, have done an Area Study and have key supplies in your house, work/school and car, the next priority are your Grab-N-Go bags. While some of the material in them duplicates what you've already prepared, the key to these bags is that they are mobile. They allow you to move out of range of a disaster or emergency if forced to.

Before you get into this and your head explodes, I'm going to break this down into two types of bags. A mild one, which is also what I recommend you at least have one of at home, and then for at work/school and in your car.

Then we'll go to the Mod/Ex which has a lot of variables depending on your Area Study as to what you will need. Do not let the Mod/Ex overwhelm you. In fact, skip it if you're going through to prepare at the Mild level. Eventually go back to Mod/Ex and take a look and perhaps acquire one or two items you think might be important. Do that every so often and eventually you will have quite a complete kit.

I'm going to cover personal items I recommend such as the survival vest (more Mod/Ex). Then go through a long list of items for GnG bags with descriptions before getting to the Mod/Ex checklist. Don't panic over the list, because you'll immediately see I'm covering a lot of gear, but in the explanation you will realize what you need and don't need. You'll see the mild bag only has a handful of items.

During my time on an A-Team, I spent a great amount of time in Isolation prior to a mission packing and repacking my gear. There were several factors behind this:
-Weight. Since we carried everything, we looked at everything we took deciding between necessity and weight. How much can you and the members on your team carry?
-Size. How much room does it take? You can only fit so much into a backpack.
-Pack your bag so you can access the most needed items first. So you have to think reverse: first in is last needed.

Optimally, we'd want to take *everything* with us. But you can't. There is no one right bag. You have to configure your GnG bag to your situation and your surrounding environment based on the area study you've already done. Prioritize depending on what you envision your survival needs being, along with the likelihood of emergencies.

Again, like almost everything else, you can buy a pre-packed GnG bag on line. These are generic, and usually packed with cheaper items to keep the cost down. For a car, I think a pre-packed bag with specific equipment for a car is an alright idea. But for your other bags, I think you should do it yourself, making it specific to your needs. Do you want to go cheap when your life depends on it?

When picking items, choose those that can have multiple uses instead of one. I have a hand crank survival radio that also has a built in flashlight and an adapter for charging my cell phone and a solar charger. Three items in one with two non-electric power sources.

Use a bag that is at least water repellant, if not waterproof. If it isn't waterproof, pack your items in waterproof bags. A key lesson of life in nature is to keep things waterproofed.

Before we get to the bags, let's move outward from your clothing.

MILD GRAB-N-GO

Personal Items

I always carry a Leatherman multi-tool on my belt. Your job/school might not allow this, but keep one close at hand; in your locker, in your desk, your purse or in your car. In the same nylon case on my belt is a small, single AAA battery, flashlight. You'll be amazed how often you use it for day-to-day activities and it can be a life-saver in a survival situation.

Always carry your cell phone. Throughout this books I reference Apps you can download and there will be a complete listing of them in Appendix B along with links. These can, literally be lifesavers.

I carry my keys attached to a credit card sized survival tool. It has a number of small tools, such as knife, compass, tweezers, etc all in one small credit card size.

Task Thirty-Five
Mild: Personal Items checklist

	Leatherman: https://amzn.to/2Cxvyry
	AAA flashlight in case with Leatherman
	Cell phone
	Credit Card Survival Tool: https://amzn.to/2CvDOYX

To go from mild personal items to Mod/Ex, a vest is useful. Hanging next to my main Grab-n-Go bag, I have what I call the emergency vest. This is similar to what members of the military wear called MOLLE gear. I use a Blackhawk Omega Crosssdraw Mag Vest, but you can also use a fishing vest, or something similar. Whatever vest has a bunch of pockets in it that can be secured.

Things to carry in it: Quikclot bandage with Israeli combat dressings.

Lighter. After many deployments and time in the field I am a firm believer in the rule that you can never have enough lighters!

Zip ties. On top of zip ties I also carry handcuff ties. Just in case. It's the easiest way to immobilize someone.

Survival knife. More on knives elsewhere. Bottom line: we're not Rambo nor do we need to be.

Ammunition for primary rifle and pistol

Compass (tied off). I like a clear compass I can lay down on the map sheet to orient it and also offset declination.

Map (tied off in case).

Task Thirty-Six
Mod/Ex: Survival Vest checklist

	Vest: https://amzn.to/2Cxvyry
	Israeli Battle Dressings: https://amzn.to/2LzJSm6
	Quikclot gauze: https://amzn.to/2BHIdXs
	Storm proof lighters: https://amzn.to/2BBC4Md
	Survival Knife: https://amzn.to/2LwgGfQ
	Compass: https://amzn.to/2GAOycI
	Map and case. Already covered.
	Assorted zip ties along with Handcuff zip ties: https://amzn.to/2Rdar61

Task Thirty-Seven
Mild: Grab-n-Go checklist

	First aid kit: https://amzn.to/2RdEc6Q
	Emergency Radio: https://amzn.to/2GCTMEJ
	Hand crank Flashlight: https://amzn.to/2Vg1bgK
	Emergency rations—one of the following **Grizzly Gear:** https://amzn.to/2Lzqk1l **ERbar:** https://amzn.to/2SfllW4 **DaTrex 3600:** https://amzn.to/2LzqtBV
	Poncho: https://amzn.to/2CxAY5G
	Water 6 bottles
	550/parachute cord: https://amzn.to/2CxSneD
	Extra keys home/car
	Extra medication
	Extra set of glasses
	Boots/workout shoes/socks

Very basic, very simple. You'd preferably be wearing the boots/workout shoes, but the concept of a GnG bag is literally that: no time and running out the door.

MOD/EX GRAB-N-GO

This list is not an absolute. You must adjust based on your environment and your Area Study. More importantly, how much will fit and you can carry on foot? Factor in what gear you can readily scavenge or make from field expediency.

The gear is broken down by areas. I explain the item, then a checklist follows. If you're uncertain what exactly the item is, you can click on the link and get an idea. Feel free to personalize, upgrade, whatever. This is a guideline.

The bag itself. This goes back to how much you can carry. Remember, the bigger the bag, the more obvious it is. And the more someone might want to steal it from you. If you have no experience with backpacks, go to your local sporting good store (REI always has knowledgeable personnel working) and ask.

Do you want just a regular backpack like kids take to school? An internal frame ruck? External frame? Built in hydrating system? The choices are limitless. What you should do is go down this list first, write out what you'd like in the bag, get the stuff, then find a bag that fits the stuff. You might find you're trying to carry too much. That's when you take out the items depending on importance. Also, consider the color of the bag. I'd go with, if not camouflage, something that is dark in color, or that matches your surrounding terrain.

WATER
4 full 500ml water bottles. This is your immediate emergency supply if you have no time to fill up your . . .

Water Containers. Either a built in water supply such as a Camelbak or pockets/clips for water carriers. Most packs have external loops on which you can secure canteens and water carriers. Remember, though, that water sloshing about and things on the outside of your bag banging about, violates noise discipline. Your first priority is to fill up this container with potable water or fill from your household water stash if bugging out. The four water bottles are to sustain you to get to that point. They also then become extra water containers.

Water Purification.

Lifestraw equivalent and two bottles purification tablets.

Water Filter

Water purifying tablets

Waterproof Sacks, inner bags, Ziploc bags. Everything inside your backpack that can get wet needs to be inside a waterproof sack/inner bag. Have a supply of assorted size Ziploc bags for smaller gear.

Empty compressible water containers: For after establishing base camp

FIRE

Windproof lighters. 3 each.

Windproof matches with striker.

Magnesium fire starter. Make sure you practice with it before trying it for the first time in the midst of a downpour and hurricane force winds.

Portable stove and fuel supply. You need a small stove with a fuel supply for at least a few days. Go with the stove for cooking initially instead of a fire because of smoke and light discipline.

FOOD

Minimum 3 days supply. Add in power bars, etc. Survival meals.

Pot to cook in, utensils, pot holder.

FIRST AID
Emergency first aid kit.
Medical mask.
Quikclot sponge. 2 each
Universal Splint, rolled. 1 each.
Extra medication (minimum one week's worth)
Extra glasses

SHELTER
Emergency, light weight sleeping bag. These are also called bivy sacks. They are a step up from the emergency blankets you see advertised and more effective.

Small tent or poncho. This depends on multiple factors: how many people, portability, weather, etc. As you'll see later, my recommendation for the hide site is to make it out of tents in a remote location. If you're hard-core, you eschew the tent in favor of a field expedient shelter that can be put up and taken down quickly, using a poncho and paracord. This also depends on the weather/Area Study.

Sleeping pad. Either a fixed pad or Thermarest self-inflating. Not just for comfort, but in cold environments, staying off the ground, saves you heat. In a hot, jungle environment, this can be swapped out for a hammock.

Insect repellent adequate for your environment

Sleeping bag*. Your decision on a sleeping bag depends on your Area Study. Plus 20? Minus 20? A bivy sack is useful for both shelter and sleeping. You need something waterproof to insert the sleeping bag into.

TOOLS
Leatherman, Mutli-Tool (in addition, consider adding Leatherman, Crunch Multi-Tool)

Portable, hand crank, emergency radio.

Hand crank rechargeable flashlight.

Battery powered headlamp. Often, in the dark, doing survival activities, you'll need both hands, so this helps. Also, consider having a red lens cover or red option for the light so you can use it at night and not emit out a large signature.

Fixed blade survival knife. We used to argue about knives all the time in our team room. Which type was best, where to carry it, etc. etc. You don't need a Rambo type knife, in fact, it's too big and too heavy. I like a six to eight inch blade with a serrated edge on the back side for sawing. With sharpening stone.

Folding saw. These are very useful in cutting firewood, clearing paths and construction.

Paracord. 100 feet at least. Parachute cord or 550 cord as we called it in the army. This is very strong, very light and narrow cord that again, will have more uses than you can imagine.

Signal mirror

Signal panel, such as a VS-17. This is why everything else is muted or camouflaged. You keep this packed away until you actually want to signal someone.

Fishing Line, hooks, sinkers and some lures. These come in handy kits.

Snare wire. Indispensable. You'll be amazed how many different uses you'll find for this beyond setting snares. Traps are a much more efficient way to catch game over hunting. Hunting with a gun also leaves a noise signature that might attract unwanted guests.

Electrical tape. 1 roll.

Duct tape. 1 roll.

Candles. Primarily in a winter environment for light, warmth, fire, glazing snow cave, etc.

Survival axe.

Machete.   If applicable to your environment and zombie threat level.

Snow shovel. If applicable to your environment

Pocket chainsaw. Light weight, small, but can be very useful in a variety of situations. Such as amputating your own arm if its pinned to a canyon wall by a boulder. Joking. Not.

MISC.

Compass.

Zip ties. An assortment. Very useful.

Map of the area. A physical, geographic map. 1:24,000 scale at least.

Waterproof Map case. Make sure there is a way to tie this off to you.

Pen, pencil and paper.

Identification. Driver's license, passport.

Weapons. Will be discussed elsewhere.

Optics. A small pair of binoculars or a small telescope could be very valuable. Some say night vision goggles but now you're crossing the line into the Apocalypse and Zombies. I don't see NVGs being in your GnG bag unless you live in Nome, Alaska where it's dark 24 hours a day and vampires can come and have a buffet as they did in *30 Days of Night.* Then get a set so you can at least see the vampire that kills you.

Cash. ATMs won't work if the power is out. Cash will be an initial barter material. This will be the initial barter material until it gets real bad when food, first aid, expertise (especially medical) and weapons/ammunition will take priority.

Apps: Load the Apps in Appendix B.

PERSONAL ITEMS

Toilet paper. Baby wipes are preferable.

Toothbrush with paste

Razor and blades
Camping soap
Camping towel (small, dries fast)
Feminine hygiene products as needed

CLOTHING

Pair of workout shoes or broken in boots, in case you have to bug out and don't have time to put on your proper bug out clothing

Extra socks. At least three pair.

Boot bands. Seems trivial, until things start crawling up your legs.

Wool watch cap. Most heat escapes through the head and/or:

Boonie hat. Protection from the sun, absorbs sweat.

Gloves. For weather as appropriate but also for working. Something that gives you a good grip while also protecting your skin. When I was in the field, I wore thin gloves pretty much all the time. They allowed me to handle my weapon but also protected my hands.

Task Thirty-Eight
Mod/Ex Grab-n-Go checklist

	WATER
	4 water bottles
	Water containers/canteens/Camelbak
	Lifestraw: https://amzn.to/2V8udyM
	Water filter: https://amzn.to/2V7PIjb
	Water purifying tablets: https://amzn.to/2LAqndh
	Waterproof sacks
	Compressible water containers: https://amzn.to/2Lzj1qC
	FIRE
	Stormproof lighters: https://amzn.to/2V8Ld87
	Windproof matches: https://amzn.to/2SkR2x9
	Magnesium fire starter: https://amzn.to/2SjWkJk
	Portable stove and fuel: https://amzn.to/2Lzj59Q
	FOOD
	3 day supply food
	Emergency rations **Grizzly Gear:** https://amzn.to/2Lzqk1l **ERbar:** https://amzn.to/2SfllW4

DaTrex 3600: https://amzn.to/2LzqtBV
Cooking pots: https://amzn.to/2SenkKs **Utensils:** https://amzn.to/2Afz0p7

	FIRST AID
	First aid kit: https://amzn.to/2RdEc6Q
	Quikclot bandage, First Aid bandage, rolled splint: https://amzn.to/2VbgcAb
	Extra medication for one week at least
	Extra glasses (old pair is better than nothing)
	SHELTER
	Emergency bivy sack: https://amzn.to/2BDuPDx
	Small tent or poncho
	550/parachute cord: https://amzn.to/2CxSneD
	Tent stakes if just using poncho
	Sleeping pad: https://amzn.to/2VbWKUf
	Sleeping bag
	Insect repellant
	CLOTHING
	Workout shoes or boots
	Extra socks
	Boot bands
	Boonie hat or wool cap
	Gloves

	TOOLS
	Emergency Radio: https://amzn.to/2GCTMEJ
	Hand crank Flashlight: https://amzn.to/2Vg1bgK
	Battery powered headlamp: https://amzn.to/2RdecZk
	Signal Mirror: https://amzn.to/2BGKOAy
	VS-17 signal panel: https://amzn.to/2Sqqzyz
	Folding Saw: https://amzn.to/2LwcHQF
	Fishing Kit: https://amzn.to/2BC36TK
	Snares: https://amzn.to/2Lwd6Tb
	Electrical tape
	Candles (per Area Study) useful for glazing snow caves
	Survival axe (per Area Study) also is a weapon: https://amzn.to/2BDuAby
	Machete (per Area Study): https://amzn.to/2CxTgE4
	Snow shovel (per Area Study): https://amzn.to/2RkYNpA
	Pocket chainsaw (per Area Study): https://amzn.to/2BI7YqC

	MISC ITEMS
	Compass: https://amzn.to/2GAOycI
	Assorted zip ties along with Handcuff zip ties: https://amzn.to/2Rdar61
	Map of Area
	Waterproof map case
	Pen, paper, pencil
	Optics (binoculars or telescope—as per Area study)
	CASH
	Apps downloaded from Appendix B
	Toilet paper
	Toothbrush and paste
	Razor and blades
	Camping soap
	Camping towel
	Feminine hygiene products as needed

In conclusion:

Lay out everything you want to put in your various GnG bags. Will it all fit? If not, prioritize what doesn't go.

When you pack the bag, pack it backwards: what is least important goes in first. What you might need right away is last in, or in outside pockets. Can you carry it? Put it on. Go for a walk. A long walk. In your survival boots. Take a walk. Cross-country. See how it feels. How it contours to your body.

Get the various bags in place: home, car, and work/school.

You have three Grab-n-Go bags ready!

We now move from Preparing into Survival.

SURVIVAL

First Five Things To Do In An Emergency

Every situation is different and this is a guideline. Always make sure your priority is safety for yourself first, then others. You can't help others if you don't take care of yourself.

First:

Do a First Aid triage of yourself. Breathing. Bleeding. Broken.

Are you stabilized?

Can you move?

Assess the immediate situation. Take charge.

If in immediate danger, get to a safe place. If you're not in immediate danger, look around.

What are the priorities of threats? Other people will be panicking. Don't get caught up in that. Be aware that any situation can get worse. In fact, assume it will. Also, having done your Area Study, you know there are after-effects of various emergencies and natural disaster. Earthquakes around the coast can lead to tsunamis. A terrorist attack could have a follow on attack for first responders. A hurricane can lead to broken gas lines which lead to a fire danger.

Check for smoke, gases and fumes. Locate and shut off the source if possible. Fires, earthquakes, bombs, etc. produce structural instability. Just because the roof is still there, doesn't mean it will stay there.

If in a car accident, turn off ignition, look out for pools of gas or any smoke.

Second:

Call for help. Dial 911. Yell. Blow a whistle. Tap on a pipe with a piece of metal. Whatever is appropriate to the event. If you're performing CPR, yell at someone nearby to call for help. Tell them what to say.

Getting trained personnel on the scene quickly is the best assistance you can render others. If you talk to a dispatcher, give a succinct summary of the situation: Location; what the emergency is; how many casualties and an estimate of condition; any potential threats.

If it is a mass casualty event, let them know that right away as the response will be different as a single responding unit would be overwhelmed.

Third:

Do a First Aid Triage of others. Triage comes from the French word 'to sort'. The goal is to rapidly assess and prioritize a number of injured individuals and do the most good for the most people. The key here is it IS NOT to do the best for *every* individual.

First, make sure the injured are not in imminent danger.

How many are injured? How badly?

Who can assist you?

Can assistance get to you?

Can the wounded by moved if they have to be? Do you have the means to move them?

If immediate help is on the way, don't take any unnecessary risks. Don't move an injured person unless they are in immediate danger. Don't treat past life-saving measures. Let the professionals do their job when they arrive. Your job is to maintain until help arrives.

What is the status of your A-Team? If some members aren't present, where are they? Can you communicate with them and arrange to meet? If you can't communicate with them, can you contact your out of area emergency contact? If that's not possible the priority of meeting locations will be in order: home, IRP, ERP.

Fourth:

Assess the environment. Can you stay or do you need to leave? Do you have adequate shelter where you are for the environment? If you're staying, at home, at the IRP, ERP, work, school, wherever, inventory your supplies and gather what you can. Focus on water, communication, food and medical.

If leaving and you have time, dress in your emergency clothing. Take your Grab-n-Go bag (home, car or work/school). If leaving, are you going to the IRP to meet A-Team? Or is it best to go direct to the ERP?

If you're leaving and not going to any of those, what is your destination? Your out of area emergency contact? Are they clear of the effect of the emergency or disaster? The destination should be chosen by priority among shelter, water, food, and medication.

Fifth:

Once in a safe place, assess the overall situation and make long term plans.

The Key Phrase: SURVIVAL

The most important tool for preparation and survival is having the right mindset. All the training, preparation, information, tools, etcetera, are useless without the will to survive. This will is birthed from having the right mindset.

Don't be intimidated. The will to survive is in every person. Luckily, for most of us, we haven't had to tap into it. But when you have to, *you will*. Human beings are amazingly adaptable. I've talked to people who say: If it's that bad, I don't want to survive. But my experience says you'll react differently. And when you do, this book will have you ready.

Here are some tools to help you:

The word ***Survival*** provides you with the first letters of the keys you need.

S - Size up the situation, your surroundings, yourself, and your equipment.

U - Use All Your Senses & Undue Haste Makes Waste

R - Remember Where You Are

V - Vanquish Fear and Panic

I - Improvise

V - Value Living

A - Act Like the Natives

L - Live by Your Wits

S: Size up the situation, your surroundings, yourself, and your equipment

There are two ways to do this: one is in preparation and the other is in the actual situation. For preparation, you sized up your potential situations by doing the Area Study.

Size up your situation: Focus on what exactly is the threat in order of priority? This might seem obvious, but consider the situation in Japan in 2011. The initial event was the earthquake. That, however, wasn't the primary threat. The resulting tsunami caused much more devastation. And following that, the problems at the nuclear plants presented immense issues that are still having an effect.

Size up your surroundings: When in a situation, tune in to the environment. Wherever you are, you are part of a system. This is key to survival. You don't want to fight your environment; you want to work with it. There is a pattern to nature. In an urban environment there are also patterns. Make note of the patterns and also focus on any time the pattern is disturbed.

One thing that always struck me was that no matter where my A-Team went in the world, no matter how hard we tried to hide, no matter how far from civilization we were, the locals always knew we were there. Because our presence was abnormal. They sensed it. Do the same with your environment.

Size up yourself: Have you, or someone on your team, been hurt or wounded? Often, in the initial rush of a trauma, we miss potentially lethal injuries. We'll discuss emergency first aid later, but you must take the time to assess everyone's physical condition. For example, with gunshot wounds, the exit wound can be more dangerous than the entrance wound, but often people don't look for it.

Keep yourself healthy. Dehydration, which we'll cover under water, is a major problem that can easily be avoided.

Notice how this is emphasized in *The Hunger Games*. The first piece of advice the mentor gives to the two candidates from his district is to find water. We can survive quite a while without food, but water is critical. Cold and wet are also enemies that you have to monitor and deal with.

Size up your equipment: What do you have? What can you get? What condition is your equipment in? What do you have that is necessary and what can you do without? During the tsunami in Japan many people died while they tried to pick up what they felt were irreplaceable items. Some people even went back to their houses after initially evacuating and died. The most important things are people, not memorabilia or jewels or money.

U - Use All Your Senses, Undue Haste Makes Waste

Use all your senses. A key trait, which mystifies many people, is called 6th sense. Great point men in the army are valued for this trait. They'll be leading a patrol along a trail and suddenly stop. Something has alerted them, but they can't pinpoint it right away. We all have 6th sense, but many of us don't pay attention to it. 6th sense is one or more of your other 5 senses picking up something real and alerting your subconscious. You actually saw or smelled or felt something, but didn't consciously register it. Trust that feeling. Focus and shift whatever it is to your conscious mind. Listen, smell, taste, touch, see. All are critical.

One of the books recommended in Appendix E is *The Gift of Fear*. It discusses this in more detail for day to day living.

Undue haste makes waste: Unless you are in imminent danger, slow down and think things through. Panic is a killer. If you don't think and plan, you could do the wrong thing and in some cases cause a 'no do-over' action, which is usually fatal. Don't take an action or move just for the sake of doing something. Every action and movement must have a purpose.

The good news is that once you finish this book and have done the task checklists you will be much more ready and will have anticipated many potential problems and be prepared for them.

R - Remember Where You Are
Know your location at all times. Also, know where the people on your team are. Stay oriented. Often you can use significant terrain features for that, whether it be a coastline, a mountain range, a river. They can also give you boundaries.

We'll go over traditional map reading later in this book because we have become overly reliant on GPS. We'll discuss maps, how to get them for free, how to use them, and field expedient direction finding techniques.

Make sure everyone in the group is oriented. Make sure you know who has the map and compass. The map is inside a waterproof case. The map and compass are tied off to your body with a 'dummy' cord. Never rely on others to know where you're located. If you are moving, make note of key terrain features and water sources. Remember, water sources are where game congregate and usually have fish in them, so they are also food sources.

During training at the International Mountain Climbing School, an experienced mountaineer told us a key to his surviving situations where others had perished: while going up the mountain, he repeatedly looked *back*. He wanted to see what it would look like when he was coming down the mountain. More people get lost and killed coming down the mountain than going up.
LOOK BACK.

V - Vanquish Fear and Panic

Courage is acting in the face of fear. We are all capable of being heroes. And it's easier to be a hero when you're prepared, which you will be.

Don't let your imagination run too far in a fatalistic direction, much like the one soldier in *Aliens* who kept screaming "We're all going to die." You don't want someone like that on your team.

Think about times in your life when you were in a crisis. How did you react? How did those people you want on your team react in a crisis? How someone reacts in a crisis gives you a very good idea of someone's core personality type in a survival situation.

Panic and fear also drain your energy. You're not focused on what needs to be done; you're focused on what could possibly go wrong. One way to help lower fear and panic is to be prepared, have a plan, and practice aspects of survival training so you build your confidence.

I - Improvise

Look at the things around you with a different mindset in a survival situation. What might have one particular use in civilization can have a very different use in a survival situation.

No matter how well prepared you are, in an extended emergency, some of your gear will wear out. How can you use other objects around you?

V - Value Living

The will to survive. You have it; tap into it.

Two men with similar, survivable wounds. One lived and one died. What was the difference? The one who lived wanted to with every atom of his being. The one who died succumbed to his fear and pain. He didn't value his life enough.

We tend to be creatures of comfort. Civilization has advanced to the point where few people have the day to day survival skills that many people had just a few generations ago. We buy our food prepared and pre-packaged. Our water comes from a tap. Electricity is taken as a given, rather than a precarious luxury. However, don't let that make you think you can't handle a survival situation.

One thing I have seen is that when people value living, they adapt surprisingly quickly. Most of our life consists of habits. When we are forced to change our habits, we rapidly adopt new ones.

No matter how hard it gets, never quit.

A - Act Like the Natives

If you are out of your natural environment, then observe those around you, both human and animal. Those that are native to the area have adapted to it. What do they eat? Where do they get their food and water? Are there places they avoid? What are their customs and habits? Remember, even customs that seem very strange, often have a very practical root.

Watching animals is key. They also need water, food and shelter. Animals can also be an alert for the presence of other humans. And they can alert others to your presence.

If you are a stranger, develop rapport with the locals. In order to get respect, you have to show respect first.

L - Live by Your Wits, But for Now, Learn Basic Skills

There are skills you need to practice, actions you need to rehearse before having to use them in an emergency. I will highlight these skills as we go through the book.

Again, preparation is the key to success, both in terms of equipment and training.

In conclusion, you will find the traits of the survivor are also the traits, in everyday, normal living, make a person successful. So you can use this book not only to prepare, but also to learn traits that will make your current environment more fruitful and positive.

S	Size up the situation, your surroundings, yourself and your equipment
U	Use all your sense and undue haste makes waste
R	Remember where you are
V	Vanquish fear and panic
I	Improvise
V	Value Living
A	Act like the natives
L	Live by your wits

First Aid

(Disclaimer: This is advice. But every situation is different.
I am not a medical expert. I am passing on what I have learned and what I've gathered from those who are.
Always get professional medical assistance.)

Survival Triage priorities:
Breathing.
Bleeding.
Broken.

Lifesaving Steps

Remain calm and do not panic. Check yourself first, then render aid to others.

Perform a rapid physical exam. Look for the cause of the injury and follow the ABCs of first aid, starting with the airway and breathing, but be discerning. A person may die from arterial bleeding more quickly than from an airway obstruction in some cases.

If you have your cell phone and power, you've already downloaded Apps which can quickly guide you to First Aid topics and even show you video of what to do along with audio instructions. Use these Apps if you can rather than trying to read instructions.

The information below is only for emergencies when no other option is available and is not the definitive word on First Aid.

First Aid Topics Covered in Order
Breathing Health Causes
                          Emergency Causes
                          Symptoms
                          Treatment—Heimlich/CPR
                          Treatment—Allergic
Reaction/Collapses Lung
     Bleeding   Symptoms of life-threatening bleeding
                          Treatment of life-threatening bleeding
                          Controlling bleeding—Pressure and
tourniquet
                          Treating open wounds
     Burns
     Shock
     Broken   Fractures (open and closed)
     Dislocations
     Sprains
     Water   Dehydration
                          Heat Stroke
     Food   Basic, plant and animal
     Cold Weather Injuries, Frostbite and Hypothermia
     Bites and Stings.   Ticks, bees, wasps, spiders,
scorpions, snakes.
     Personal Hygeine

BREATHING

Since we can only survive three minutes without oxygen, breathing is a priority.

Difficulty breathing is always a medical emergency.

Health causes can be:

Anemia (low red blood cell count)

Asthma

Chronic obstructive pulmonary disease (COPD), more commonly called emphysema or chronic bronchitis.

Heart disease or failure.

Lung cancer, or cancer that has spread to the lungs.

Respiratory infections, including pneumonia, acute bronchitis, whooping cough, croup and others.

Pericardial effusion (fluid surrounding the heart, including blood, that won't allow it to fill properly).

Pleural effusion (fluid surround the lungs, including blood, that compresses them).

Emergency Causes of breathing problems:

Being at high altitude.

Blood clot in lungs.

Pneumothorax (collapsed lung).

Heart attack.

Injury to the neck, chest wall, or lungs.

Foreign matter in mouth or throat that obstructs the opening to the trachea.

Inflammation and swelling of mouth and throat caused by inhaling smoke, flames, and irritating vapors or by an allergic reaction.

Kink in the throat (caused by the neck bent forward so that the chin rests upon the chest) may block the passage of air.

Tongue blocks passage of air to the lungs upon unconsciousness. When an individual is unconscious, the muscles of the lower jaw and tongue relax as the neck drops forward, causing the lower jaw to sag and the tongue to drop back and block the passage of air.

Life-threatening allergic reaction.

Near drowning, with fluid build up in the lungs.

Symptoms:

Rapid breathing.

Unable to breathe lying down and needing to sit up to breathe.

Very anxious or agitated.

Sleepy or confused.

Dizziness.

Coughing.

Nausea.

Vomiting.

Bluish lips, fingers and fingernails.

Chest moving in an unusual way.

Gurgling, wheezing or whistling sounds.

Difficulty speaking or muffled voice.

Coughing up blood.

Rapid or irregular heartbeat.

If an allergy is causing the problem, there might be a rash or swelling of the face, tongue, or throat.

If an injury is causing the problem, there might be bleeding or a visible wound.

Treatment:

A key to remember is that leaning the head back opens the airway in the throat as much as possible.

You can open an airway and maintain it by using the following steps.

Step 1. Check if the victim has a partial or complete airway obstruction. If he can cough or speak, allow him to clear the obstruction naturally. Stand by, reassure the victim, and be ready to clear his airway and perform mouth-to-mouth resuscitation should he become unconscious. If his airway is completely obstructed, administer the Heimlich until the obstruction is cleared.

Step 2. Using a finger, quickly sweep the victim's mouth clear of any foreign objects, broken teeth, dentures, sand, dirt, etc.

Step 3. Using the jaw thrust method, grasp the angles of the victim's lower jaw and lift with both hands, one on each side, moving the jaw forward. For stability, rest your elbows on the surface on which the victim is lying. If his lips are closed, gently open the lower lip with your thumb. *Lean the head back to further open the airway.*

Step 4. With the victim's airway open, pinch his nose closed with your thumb and forefinger and blow two complete breaths into his lungs. Allow the lungs to deflate after the second inflation and perform the following:

Look for his chest to rise and fall.

Listen for escaping air during exhalation. *Feel* for flow of air on your cheek.

Step 5. If the forced breaths do not stimulate spontaneous breathing, maintain the victim's breathing by performing mouth-to-mouth resuscitation.

Step 6. There is danger of the victim vomiting during mouth-to-mouth resuscitation. Check the victim's mouth periodically for vomit and clear as needed.

Note: Cardiopulmonary resuscitation (CPR) may be necessary after cleaning the airway, but only after major bleeding is under control.

SELF HEIMLICH

Try to cough object up. If you cannot get it out, you must act quickly, before you lose consciousness.

Make a fist. Place it on your abdomen just above your navel and *below* your ribcage.

Hold the fist with your other hand for leverage.

Drive your fist in and up. Use a quick j-shaped motion. Repeat.

If the object does not dislodge, quickly find a stable, waist high object, such as the back of a chair, a table, or a counter-top. With your hands still in place, bend over it, brace your hands. Drive your body against the object.

Repeat until the object dislodges.

CHOKING—OTHER—HEIMLICH ADULT

From behind, wrap your arms around the victim's waist.

Make a fist and place the thumb side of your fist against the victim's upper abdomen, below the ribcage and above the navel.

Grasp your fist with your other hand and press into their upper abdomen with a quick upward thrust. Do not squeeze the ribcage; confine the force of the thrusts to your hands.

Repeat until the object has been expelled.

CHOKING--INFANT

Lay the child down, face up, on a firm surface.

Kneel or stand at the victim's feet, or hold the victim on your lap, facing away from you.

Place the middle and index fingers of both your hands below his rib cage and above navel.

Press in with a quick upward thrust. *Do not squeeze the rib cage*. Be gentle.

Repeat until object is expelled.

PERFORMING CPR:

(Remember you have an app to assist!)

Check the victim for responsiveness. If not responsive or not breathing or not breathing normally, call 911. Place the phone next to the victim and put in speaker mode. If necessary, in most places, the dispatcher can help you with instructions.

If the victim still is not breathing normally, coughing, or moving, begin chest compressions. Push down on the center of the chest 2 to 2.5 inches, 30 times. Pump hard and fast at the rate faster than one per second. After 30:

Tilt the head back and lift the chin. Pinch the nose and cover the mouth with yours. Blow until you see the chest rise. Do this 2 times. Each breath should take 1 second.

Go back to 30 compressions.

2 breaths.

Continue until help arrives.

If doing two person CPR, the person compressing stops while the other person gives the 2 breaths.

Treatment Allergic Reaction/Collapsed Lung:

Dealing with a Severe Allergic Reaction leading to Anaphylaxis:

Call 911 immediately.

See if they have epinephrine auto injector and use as the instructions indicate.

Keep them calm.

Have them lie on their back.

Raise their feet 12 inches and cover with a blanket.

Turn them on their side if they are vomiting or bleeding.

Make sure their clothing is loose.

Dealing with a Collapsed Lung:

A collapsed lung can be caused several ways including:

A puncture from a broken rib.

A puncture wound through the chest wall (a sucking chest wound).

A weak part of the lung that starts leaking.

Signs and symptoms:

Sudden pain on the affected side.

Shortness of breath.

Obvious wound to the chest.

If you have a stethoscope you can listen on that side of the chest and breath sounds are either absent or greatly decreased.

Treatment:

If it's a puncture wound and the object is still in place, leave it in place and call for help or get assistance.

If it's an open sucking chest wound allowing air in to the lung, bandage the wound, using an airproof material or bandage first, such as plastic wrap, a plastic bag, or gauze pads covered with petroleum jelly, sealing it, except for one corner, allowing air to escape, but not go in.

Do not give the person food or drink.

Do not move the person unless absolutely necessary.

Do not place anything under their head to raise it as this will restrict the air passage.

Do not wait to see if their condition improves before getting help.

BLEEDING

An average adult weighing between 150 and 180 pounds, has about 4.7 to 5.5 liters, or 1.2 to 1.5 gallons (5 to 6 quarts) of blood.

Losing 1 liter, or 1 quart, of blood will begin to send someone into shock. Losing 2 liters, 2 quarts, will induce severe shock. Losing 3 liters, 3 quarts, usually results in death.

Symptoms of life-threatening bleeding are:
Spurting blood.

Blood that won't stop.

Blood that is pooling on the ground.

Clothing that is soaked with blood.

Bandages that are soaked with blood.

Loss of all or part of a leg or arm.

Continued bleeding in a victim who is confused and unconscious.

Treatment of life-threatening bleeding:
The key is to find and compress the bleeding blood vessel to stop the flow of blood.

Find the source of the bleeding. Remove clothing from over the wound.

Apply pressure. Any cloth will do, but if you have the Quikclot you should have, that will help. If the wound is deep, stuff the cloth/bandage into the wound.

Put a compression bandage on the wound, if available. Push down as hard as you can.

If a compression bandage is not available, apply continuous pressure until help arrives.

Tourniquet
For life-threatening bleeding from an arm or leg and the above doesn't work.

Wrap the tourniquet around the limb 2 to 3 inches above the source of the blood. Do NOT put it on a joint. Go above the joint if necessary.

Pull the free end of the tourniquet as tight as possible and then secure it around a solid stick or rod (windlass).

Note the time it was applied.

Controlling Bleeding:
In a survival situation, you must control serious bleeding immediately because replacement fluids (IVs) are usually not available and the victim can die within a matter of minutes. External bleeding falls into the following classifications:

Arterial. Blood vessels called arteries carry blood away from the heart and through the body. A cut artery issues *bright red* blood from the wound in *distinct spurts* or pulses that correspond to the rhythm of the heartbeat. Because the blood in the arteries is under high pressure, an individual can lose a large volume of blood in a short period when there is damage to an artery. Therefore, arterial bleeding is the most serious type of bleeding. If not controlled promptly, it can be fatal.

Venous. Venous blood is blood that is returning to the heart through blood vessels called veins. A steady flow of *dark red, maroon, or bluish* blood characterizes bleeding from a vein.

Capillary. The capillaries are the extremely small vessels that connect the arteries with the veins. Capillary bleeding most commonly occurs in minor cuts and scrapes.

You can control external bleeding by direct pressure, elevation, digital ligation, or tourniquet.

Direct Pressure

The most effective way to control external bleeding is by applying pressure directly over the wound. This pressure must not only be firm enough to stop the bleeding, but it must also be maintained long enough to allow the bleeding to stop on its own.

Using a Quikclot bandage can help greatly.

If bleeding continues after having applied direct pressure for 30 minutes, apply a pressure dressing. This dressing consists of a thick dressing of gauze, a Quikclot sponge, or other suitable material applied directly over the wound and held in place with a tightly wrapped bandage or tape. It should be tighter than an ordinary compression bandage but not so tight that it impairs circulation to the rest of the limb if on an appendage. Once you apply the dressing, *do not remove it,* even when the dressing becomes blood soaked. If blood continues to come through, though, then you have a more serious problem. If bleeding stops, leave the pressure dressing in place for at least a day, after which you can carefully remove it and replace it with a smaller dressing.

In a long-term emergency, change bandages every day and inspect for signs of infection.

Signs a wound is infected:

Expanding redness around the wound, including red streaks.

Running a fever.

Fluid draining that is cloudy or yellow/green pus or the wound is foul-smelling.

Increasing tenderness, swelling or pain around the wound.

Elevation

Raising an injured extremity as high as possible above the level of the heart slows blood loss by aiding the return of blood to the heart and lowering the blood pressure at the wound. However, elevation alone *will not* control bleeding entirely; you must also apply direct pressure over the wound. If treating a snakebite, however, keep the extremity lower than the heart.

Tourniquet

Use a tourniquet on a limb only when direct pressure over the bleeding point and all other methods did not control the bleeding. If you leave a tourniquet in place too long, the damage to the tissues can progress to gangrene, with a loss of the limb. An improperly applied tourniquet can also cause permanent damage to nerves and other tissues at the site of the constriction.

What can you use for a field expedient tourniquet? Use something that is at least 1 inch wide out to 2 inches. Using something like parachute cord or string, that is too narrow and can cut into the skin. A pressure cuff can loosen. Using something too wide will make it too hard to tighten down. A belt is good. There are commercially available tourniquets, such as a CAT (Combat Application Tourniquet-- http://amzn.to/2gZEkF4 available for less than $20 at Amazon).

If you must use a tourniquet, place it around the extremity, between the wound and the heart, 2 to 4 inches above the wound site. Never place it directly over the wound or a fracture or a joint. Use a stick as a handle to tighten the tourniquet and tighten it only enough to stop blood flow. When you have tightened the tourniquet, securely bind the free end of the stick to the limb to prevent unwinding.

After you secure the tourniquet, clean and bandage the wound.

If you've applied this to yourself and you are alone, do not remove or release. You could lose too much blood in the process and pass out, then bleed out. In a buddy system, however, the buddy can release the tourniquet pressure every 10 to 15 minutes for 1 or 2 minutes to allow blood flow to the rest of the extremity to prevent limb loss.

Dangers of using a tourniquet:

Applying too loosely. This can cause bleeding to worsen as the venous (return) blood is blocked because it is under less pressure, but arterial blood still bleeds out.

Releasing it too soon, causing severe bleeding to resume. Also, this could cause venous blood to damage compressed blood vessels.

Leaving it on too long, causing neurovascular damage and tissue death. Permanent nerve, muscle and blood vessel damage occurs after about two hours. If the choice is between this and bleeding out, then go with keeping alive.

Periodic loosening could lead to the victim bleeding out. This is a damned if you do, damned if you don't scenario.

Applying a tourniquet to a victim with low blood pressure who is in shock or receiving CPR. If the person is revived, their bleeding will increase as blood pressure increases.

Open Wounds

If the bleeding has stopped, you must now treat an open wound. Beyond the problem of the tissue damage and blood loss, there is the great concern of infection. In a high moderate to extreme emergency, the lack of access to medical care makes infections a life-threatening situation. Better to prevent them, than have to deal with them.

Infection comes from dirt on the object that made the wound, on the individual's skin and clothing, or on other foreign material or dirt that touches the wound.

By taking proper care of the wound you can reduce further contamination and promote healing.

Clean the wound as soon as possible after it occurs by:
Remove or cut clothing away from the wound.

Always looking for an exit wound if a sharp object, gun shot, or projectile caused the wound.

Thoroughly cleaning the skin around the wound.

Rinse (not scrub) the wound with sterile water.

The open treatment method is the safest way to manage wounds in survival situations. Do not try to close the wound by suturing or similar procedures. Leave the wound open to allow the drainage of any pus resulting from infection.

Cover the wound with a clean dressing. Place a bandage on the dressing to hold it in place. Change the dressing daily to check for infection.

To treat an infected wound:

Place a warm, moist compress directly on the infected wound. Change the compress when it cools, keeping a warm compress on the wound for a total of 30 minutes. Apply the compresses three or four times daily.

Drain the wound. Open and gently probe the infected wound with a sterile instrument.

Dress and bandage the wound. Drink a lot of water.

Continue this treatment daily until all signs of infection have disappeared.

If you do not have antibiotics and the wound has become severely infected, does not heal, and ordinary debridement is impossible, consider maggot therapy, despite its hazards:

Expose the wound to flies for one day and then cover it.

Check daily for maggots. Once maggots develop, keep the wound covered but check daily. Remove all maggots when they have cleaned out all dead tissue and before they start on healthy tissue. Increased pain and bright red blood in the wound indicate that the maggots have reached healthy tissue. Flush the wound repeatedly with sterile water to remove the maggots. Check the wound every four hours for several days to ensure all maggots have been removed. Bandage the wound and treat it as any other wound.

Shock
Shock is a life-threatening medical condition resulting from an insufficient flow of blood throughout the body. It can lead to other conditions such as lack of oxygen in the body's tissues (hypoxia), heart attack, or organ damage. If not treated, it can kill. Once shock sets in, unless treated, it will get worse quickly.

In an emergency situation, without immediate aid, people with survivable wounds and injuries can die from shock.

It's beyond the scope of this book, but having a trained person on your team who can administer IVs is a great boon. In Special Forces we trained on giving each other and even ourselves IVs.

Symptoms of shock:
Cold, clammy skin.
Pale, ashen skin.
Confusion and lack of alertness.
Rapid pulse.
Nausea or vomiting.
Enlarged pupils.
Weakness or fatigue.
Loss of consciousness.

Prevent and Treat Shock
If the victim is conscious, place on a level surface with the legs and feet elevated slightly.

If the victim is unconscious, place him on his side or abdomen with his head turned to one side to prevent choking on vomit, blood, or other fluids.

Once the victim is in a shock position, do not move him.

Maintain body heat by using blankets, coats, whatever is at hand.

If the person is wet, remove the wet clothing as soon as possible and replace with dry.

If conscious, and other wounds do not preclude, slowly administer small doses of a warm salt or sugar solution. If unconscious or there is an abdominal wound, do not administer fluids.

Have them rest for at least a day to recover.

If it's you, and you are alone, get to a shelter, and rest with feet slightly elevated.

BROKEN—BONE & JOINT INJURIES

Bone and joint injuries include fractures, dislocations, and sprains.

Fractures

There are two types of fractures: open and closed. With an open (or compound) fracture, the bone protrudes through the skin and complicates the actual fracture with an open wound. After setting the fracture, treat the wound as any other open wound unless there is arterial bleeding. Stopping the bleeding is then the priority. A closed fracture has no open wounds and the skin is intact. Follow the guidelines for immobilization, and set and splint the fracture.

Symptoms:

Swelling or bruising over a bone.

Deformity of an arm or leg.

Pain in the area that gets worse when the area is moved or pressure is applied.

Loss of function in the injured area.

In compound fractures, bone protruding from the skin.

There could be grating (sound and/or feeling when two ends rub together).

Treatment:

As with any other injury, optimally you would stabilize the victim until proper treatment or evacuation by trained professionals.

Move the broken limb as little as possible. A danger is that the broken ends of the bone could cut a blood vessel causing internal bleeding leading to shock and ultimately death. Moving the broken ends could also cause nerve damage. If the area below the break becomes numb, swollen, cool to the touch, or turns pale, and the victim shows signs of shock, a major vessel may have been severed. Treat the victim for shock, and replace lost fluids.

Only try to reset the break as a last resort and if help is not on the way and you are isolated.

To set the break, you are trying to relieve pain and return the limb to its anatomically correct position. This is called traction. You hold upper part of the limb above the break in place, and put tension on the lower part, lining them up. If alone, you can wedge a foot or hand, and then use the other limb to push against whatever you are wedged in.

Once you set the break, you have to maintain the position with a splint. You should have one in your Grab-n-Go bag. If not, use anything long and solid, such as branches.

Put these on either side of the break. If it is an open fracture, keep them away from the open wound. Then securely tie in place.

For a broken leg:

Very strong muscles hold a broken thighbone (femur) in place making it difficult to maintain traction during healing. You can make an improvised traction splint using natural material as follows:

Get two forked branches or saplings at least 5 centimeters in diameter. Measure one from the patient's armpit to 7 to 10 inches past the unbroken leg. Measure the other from the groin to 7 to 10 inches past the unbroken leg. Ensure that both extend an equal distance beyond the end of the leg.

Pad the two splints. Notch the ends without forks and lash a 7 to 10 inch cross member made from a 5-centimeter diameter branch between them.

Using available material tie the splint around the upper portion of the body and down the length of the broken leg. Follow the splinting guidelines.

With available material, fashion a wrap that will extend around the ankle, with the two free ends tied to the cross member.

Place a 4 inch by 1 inch stick in the middle of the free ends of the ankle wrap between the cross member and the foot. Using the stick, twist the material to make the traction easier.

Continue twisting until the broken leg is as long or slightly longer than the unbroken leg.

Lash the stick to maintain traction.

Over time you may lose traction because the material weakens. Check the traction periodically. If you must change or repair the splint, maintain the traction manually for a short time.

If the fracture is an open wound, but not arterial, make sure you apply pressure and stop the bleeding.

Dislocations

A dislocation occurs in a bone joint when the bones go out of proper alignment. This tends to be very painful. It can also cause an impairment of nerve or circulatory function below the area affected.

Symptoms:
Visible deformity in the joint.
Swollen or discolored.
Intensely painful.
Immovable.
Limited range of motion.
Treatment:

Sometimes it is difficult to tell if it is a dislocation or a broken bone, so be aware of the dangers. Only try to set if there is no other choice.

To set the bones back into proper alignment you can use several methods, but manual traction or the use of weights to pull the bones are the safest and easiest. Once performed, traction decreases the victim's pain and allows for normal function and circulation. Without an X ray, you can judge proper alignment by the look and feel of the joint and by comparing it to the joint on the opposite side.

Immobilization is splinting the dislocation after traction. You can use any field-expedient material for a splint or you can splint an extremity to the body.

The basic guidelines for splinting are:

Splint above and below the fracture site.

Pad splints to reduce discomfort.

Check circulation below the fracture after making each tie on the splint.

To rehabilitate the dislocation, remove the splints after 7 to 14 days. Gradually use the injured joint until fully healed.

Sprains

A sprain is the overstretching of a tendon or ligament. They vary in severity.

Symptoms:

One of the most common joints to sprain is the ankle. This is also the most dangerous in an emergency situation as it reduces mobility. To deduce if you have a sprained ankle or a broken one:

Was there a sound/feeling when it happened? If there was an audible crack, you've got a broken bone. If there was a pop, it's likely a sprain.

Is the ankle deformed or crooked? Most likely broken.

Is the ankle numb? Most likely broken.

If you cannot move the ankle at all and/or cannot put any weight on it? Broken.

Treatment:

When treating sprains, think RICE:

R - Rest injured area.

I - Ice for 24 hours, then heat after that.

C - Compression-wrapping and/or splinting to help stabilize. If possible, leave the boot on a sprained ankle unless circulation is compromised.

E - Elevation of the affected area.

WATER AND HEAT FIRST AID

Since we can last only three days without water, it's important to understand some basics about our body and water.

Symptoms of dehydration are:

Dark urine with a very strong odor. This is the one leaders must be on the lookout for.

Low urine output.

Dark, sunken eyes.

Fatigue

Emotional instability.

To check for dehydration look for loss of skin elasticity. Pinch the skin on the back of your hand and pull it up. It should immediately go back into place. If it maintains the pinched shape for a couple of seconds, then slowly settles back, you may be dehydrated.

Delayed capillary refill in fingernail beds.

Trench line down center of tongue.

Thirst. Last on the list because you are already 2 percent dehydrated by the time you crave fluids.

Treatment:

Replace the water as you lose it. Trying to make up a deficit is difficult in an emergency situation, and thirst is not a sign of how much water you need.

Most people cannot comfortably drink more than 1 liter of water at a time. Nor do you want to. So, even when not thirsty, drink small amounts of water at regular intervals each hour to prevent dehydration.

Drink sufficient water but don't overdo it. *Over-hydration* is a potentially fatal condition. You could drink too much water for your kidneys to process. It's not just the amount, but how quickly you drink the water. Drinking too much water, too quickly, increases the amount of water in your blood. This dilutes the electrolytes, especially sodium. Sodium is critical in balancing the fluid inside and outside of cells. When there is an imbalance from over-hydration, sodium moves inside the cells, causing them to swell. This is particularly dangerous to your brain cells.

Thus one of the first symptoms is a headache. Nausea and vomiting are also symptoms. If it gets worse, more symptoms follow, including high blood pressure, confusion, double vision, drowsiness, difficulty breathing, muscle weakness and cramping. If not caught in time, seizures will occur, brain damage, coma and even death.

A dangerous thing about hyponatremia (what this is called) is that it can be confused with dehydration and people can force the victim to drink more water. Extreme sports athletes are at risk for this, as well people during a heat wave. Without access to special medications, primary treatment for this is to stop the water intake.

If you are under physical and mental stress or subject to severe conditions, increase your water intake. Drink enough liquids to maintain a urine output of at least half a quart every 24 hours.

With the loss of water there is also a loss of electrolytes (body salts). The average diet can usually keep up with these losses but in an extreme situation or illness, additional sources need to be provided. A mixture of 0.25

teaspoon of salt to 1 liter of water will provide a concentration that the body tissues can readily absorb.

Make sure you drink water while eating. This aids in digestion. In adverse conditions, particularly cold and wet environments, a leader must force his or her people to drink water, even when they don't feel like it.

Of all the First Aid problems encountered in a survival situation, the loss of water is the most preventable. Acquiring water is a different problem, one we will deal with shortly.

Dehydration Treatment:

For dehydration that is short of heat stroke:

Drink two quarts of water, juice or sports drinks in 2 to 4 hours, not all at once. Small sips every few minutes work best.

If vomiting, try ice chips, popsicles and small sips.

If also suffering from diarrhea, stay away from using sports drinks as the sugar can make it worse.

Heat Stroke

The breakdown of the body's heat regulatory system causes a heat stroke. It occurs when your core body temperature goes to 104 degrees. Other heat injuries, such as cramps or dehydration, do not always precede a heatstroke.

Heat stroke is extremely dangerous. As with all other dangerous conditions, call 911, evacuate or get profession help if possible. Heat stroke can kill or cause serious damage to the brain and other organs. It happens after prolonged exposure to high temperatures in combination with dehydration.

Symptoms:

Swollen, beet-red face.

Reddened whites of eyes.

Victim not sweating. Red, hot and dry skin.

Unconsciousness or delirium, which can cause pallor, a bluish color to lips and nail beds (cyanosis), and cool skin.

Treatment:

Fan air over the victim while wetting skin with water.

Apply ice packs to the armpits, groin, neck, and back. These areas have more blood vessels on average, so cooling them can reduce the body temperature.

Immerse the patient in a shower or tub of cool water. Or a stream or lake.

Be sure to wet the victim's head. Heat loss through the scalp is great.

Expect, during cooling:

Vomiting.

Diarrhea.

Struggling.

Shivering.

Shouting.

Prolonged unconsciousness.

Rebound heatstroke within 48 hours.

Cardiac arrest; be ready to perform CPR.

COLD WEATHER INJURIES

Hypothermia

This occurs when the body's core temperature falls to 95 degrees F or cooler. It is the opposite of heat stroke. Wind chill multiplies the effect of cold. Wind chill is the effect of moving air on exposed flesh. Wind always exacerbates the situation, which is why your outer garment should not only be water resistant, but wind resistant. A key in building shelter is to get out of the wind.

Here is a handy chart showing the effect of wind chill.

Wind Chill Chart

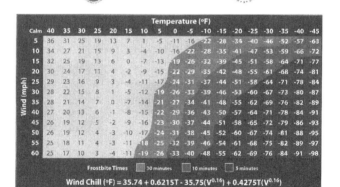

Getting wet accelerates the onset of progression of hypothermia since the body loses heat 25 times faster in cold water than in cold air. Since it changes the core temperature this means that the brain, heart, lungs and other vital organs are affected.

Some people are more susceptible to hypothermia: the elderly, children, and those under the influence of alcohol. Children and thin people lose body heat more quickly.

Cold Water Survival Times

Water Temperature	Becomes Unconscious
32.5 F	Under 15 minutes
32.5 to 40 F	15 to 30 minutes
40 to 50 F	30 to 60 minutes
50 to 60 F	1 to 2 hours
60 to 70 F	2 to 7 hours
70 to 80 F	3 to 12 hours

As you can see, even relatively mild water temperatures of 70 to 80 F can cause hypothermia. While those times are for immersion, getting wet and not being to get dry or to a shelter also causes hypothermia. As does simply staying cold even if you're not wet.

Prevention:

Avoid getting wet!

Stay hydrated.

Stay fueled; eat properly with sufficient calories for the energy expended. In Winter Warfare training, we upped our rations, knowing what we would be facing.

Seek shelter. Get out of the elements if possible. This is a situation where shelter can become more important than water or food, as being hypothermic outdoors for 3 hours can kill.

In your Grab-n-Go bag you have a wool hat and gloves. You lose 40 to 45 percent of body heat from an unprotected head and even more from the unprotected neck, wrist, and ankles. These areas of the body are good radiators of heat and have very little insulating fat.

Avoid sweating in a cold weather environment. That's causing yourself to become wet.

Symptoms:

Shivering. Confusion. Uncoordinated actions.

Treatment:

Get into shelter.

Build a fire.

Remove wet clothing and replace with dry or get in a sleeping bag or cover with blankets. Have someone who is not hypothermic share it, to give their body heat.

Sip on a warm beverage (nothing with caffeine or alcohol).

Do gentle exercises.

If you have hand warmers, put them in the same place ice would go for heat stroke: neck, armpits and groin.

Frostbite

Frostbite is the freezing of your external blood vessels and the flesh surrounding them. The most common places for this to occur are exposed skin in the ears, nose and cheeks. Also, toes, feet, fingers and hands.

Prevention: Proper clothing, worn correctly in layers, as described earlier.

Wearing gloves all the time.

Use a buddy system to check each other for symptoms.

Maintain circulation by twitching and wrinkling the skin on your face by making faces. Warm your hands. If outdoors in cold weather for an extended period of time, men shouldn't shave. Doing so removes natural oils that protect the skin.

Wiggle and move your ears. Move your hands inside your gloves. Warm by placing your hands close to your body.

Move your feet and wiggle your toes inside your boots. Change your socks often to keep them dry and clean.

Symptoms:

Stinging pain that turns into numbness. You might not even feel the pain, depending on the circumstances and what else is going on in an emergency.

The skin becomes cold to the touch and white spots develop.

Treatment:

As with everything else, medical attention ASAP; frostbite can cause permanent injuries and even amputation.

If medical attention isn't available within the next two to three hours, get into shelter and/or build a fire. Submerge body parts in water that is between 104 and 108 F; tepid water, not hot. Submerging in hot water will cause extreme pain and even shock. Do not expose frostbite to flame. This tepid water will cool quickly, drawing the cold from the body. Change it often.

When drying frostbite injuries pat them. Don't rub. Rubbing causes more damage.

Blisters may appear. Do not pop or lance them as that increases the chances of infection. Apply a loose sterile dressing over the affected area.

BITES AND STINGS

Insects and related pests are hazards in everyday life, not just emergency situations. They often carry disease. In some cases, bites and stings can be fatal because of poison or a severe allergic reactions in some individuals.

Ticks can carry and transmit diseases, such as Rocky Mountain spotted fever common in many parts of the United States. Ticks also transmit Lyme disease.

Mosquitoes may carry malaria, dengue, and other diseases.

Flies can spread disease from contact with infectious sources. They are causes of sleeping sickness, typhoid, cholera, and dysentery.

Fleas can transmit plague.

Lice can transmit typhus and relapsing fever.

The best way to avoid the complications of insect bites and stings is to keep immunizations (including booster shots) up-to-date, avoid insect-infested areas, use netting and insect repellent, and wear all clothing properly.

If you get bitten or stung, do not scratch the bite or sting, it might become infected. Inspect your body at least once a day. If you find ticks attached to your body, use tweezers to remove. Take care to remove the whole tick. Do not squeeze the tick's body. Wash your hands after doing this. Clean and disinfect the tick wound daily until healed. The old home remedy of covering the tick with petroleum jelly, fingernail polish or using a hot match are not recommended.

Bee and Wasp Stings

If stung by a bee, immediately remove the stinger and venom sac, if attached, by scraping with a fingernail or a knife blade. Do not squeeze or grasp the stinger or venom sac, as squeezing will force more venom into the wound.

Wash the sting site thoroughly with soap and water to lessen the chance of a secondary infection.

If you are allergic, you should always have your EpiPen auto-injector with you.

Spider Bites and Scorpion Stings

The black widow spider is identified by a red hourglass on its abdomen. Only the female bites and it has a neurotoxic venom. The initial pain is not severe, but severe local pain rapidly develops. The pain gradually spreads over the entire body and settles in the abdomen and legs. Abdominal cramps and progressive nausea, vomiting, and a rash may occur. Weakness, tremors, sweating, and salivation may occur. Anaphylactic reactions can occur. Symptoms begin to regress after several hours and are usually gone in a few days.

Threat for shock. Be ready to perform CPR. Clean and dress the bite area to reduce the risk of infection. An antivenom is available.

The brown house spider or brown recluse spider is a small, light brown spider identified by a dark brown violin on its back. You usually are not aware you've been bitten at the time because there is little pain. Within a few hours a painful red area with a mottled center appears. Necrosis does not occur in all bites, but usually in 3 to 4 days, a star-shaped, firm area of deep purple discoloration appears at the bite site. The area turns dark and mummified in a week or two. The margins separate and the scab falls off, leaving an open ulcer. Secondary infection and regional swollen lymph glands usually become visible at this stage. The outstanding characteristic of the brown recluse bite is an ulcer that does not heal but persists for weeks or months. In addition to the ulcer, there is often a systemic reaction that is serious and may lead to death. Speaking from experience, a brown recluse bite goes un-noticed, but eventually is painful and noticeable.

Reactions (fever, chills, joint pain, vomiting, and a generalized rash) occur chiefly in children or debilitated persons.

Scorpions are all poisonous to a greater or lesser degree. There are two different reactions, depending on the species: Severe local reaction only, with pain and swelling around the area of the sting. Possible prickly sensation around the mouth and a thick-feeling tongue.

Severe systemic reaction, with little or no visible local reaction. Local pain may be present. Systemic reaction includes respiratory difficulties, thick-feeling tongue, body spasms, drooling, gastric distention, double vision, blindness, involuntary rapid movement of the eyeballs, involuntary urination and defecation, and heart failure. Death is rare, occurring mainly in children and adults with high blood pressure or illnesses.

Snakebites

The chance of a snakebite in an emergency situation is rather small, if you are familiar with the various types of snakes and their habitats. However, it could happen and you should know how to treat a snakebite. Deaths from snakebites are rare. More than one-half of snakebite victims have little or no poisoning, and only about one-quarter develop serious systemic poisoning.

The primary concern in the treatment of snakebite is to limit the amount of eventual tissue destruction around the bite area.

A bite wound, regardless of the type of animal that inflicted it, can become infected from bacteria in the animal's mouth. With nonpoisonous as well as poisonous snakebites, this local infection is responsible for a large part of the residual damage that results.

Snake venoms not only contain poisons that attack the victim's central nervous system (neurotoxins) and blood circulation (hemotoxins), but also digestive enzymes (cytotoxins) to aid in digesting their prey. These poisons can cause a very large area of tissue death, leaving a large open wound. This condition could lead to the need for eventual amputation if not treated.

Shock and panic in a person bitten by a snake can also affect the person's recovery. Excitement, hysteria, and panic can speed up the circulation, causing the body to absorb the toxin quickly. Signs of shock could occur within the first 30 minutes after the bite.

Before you start treating a snakebite, determine whether the snake was poisonous or nonpoisonous. There are four types of poisonous snakes in North America. In your Area Study you should have determined if any are endemic to your area.

Overall, venomous snakes have a triangular head (not so much on the Coral), while non-venomous have more spoon-shaped heads.

Cottonmouths: elliptical pupils and range in color from black to green. They have a white stripe along the sides of their head. They are normally found in or around water. The young have a bright yellow tail. They usually are alone.

Rattlesnakes: A triangular head with elliptical eyes. And of course, a rattle on their tail.

Copperheads: Brightly colored from coppery brown to bright orange, silver-pink and peach. The young also have yellow tails.

Coral snakes: Several non-venomous snakes look like Coral snakes. They have a distinctive coloring, with black, yellow, and red bands. They have a yellow head with a black band over their nose. They are extremely shy and rarely bite.

The difference between a Coral and a King Snake is: "red on black, venom lack. Red on yellow, deadly fellow."

Bites from a nonpoisonous snake will show rows of teeth. Bites from a poisonous snake may have rows of teeth showing, but will have one or more distinctive puncture marks caused by fang penetration.

Symptoms of a poisonous bite may be spontaneous bleeding from the nose and anus, blood in the urine, pain at the site of the bite, and swelling at the site of the bite within a few minutes or up to 2 hours later.

Breathing difficulty, paralysis, weakness, twitching, and numbness are also signs of neurotoxic venoms. These signs usually appear 1.5 to 2 hours after the bite.

If you determine that a poisonous snake bit an individual, take the following steps:

Reassure the victim and keep him still.

Remove watches, rings, bracelets, or other constricting items.

Clean the bite area.

Maintain an airway (especially if bitten near the face or neck) and be prepared to administer mouth-to-mouth resuscitation or CPR.

Use a constricting band between the wound and the heart. Immobilize the site.

Remove the poison as soon as possible by using a mechanical suction device or by squeezing.

Do not give the victim alcoholic beverages or tobacco products.

Do not give morphine or other central nervous system (CNS) depressors.

Do not make any deep cuts at the bite site.

Do not put your hands on your face or rub your eyes, as venom may be on your hands. Venom may cause blindness.

Do not break open the large blisters that form around the bite site.

After caring for the victim as described above, take the following actions to minimize local effects:

If infection appears, keep the wound open and clean.

Use heat after 24 to 48 hours to help prevent the spread of local infection. Heat also helps to draw out an infection.

Keep the wound covered with a dry, sterile dressing.

Have the victim drink large amounts of fluids until the infection is gone.

Snakes usually avoid people. Rattlers never really concerned me; we used to eat them and they do taste like chicken. Where snakes can be dangerous is in the water. Hitting a nest of water moccasins can be deadly.

PERSONAL HYGEINE

During a high moderate or extreme emergency, you might go weeks, months and longer in uncomfortable circumstances, whether in the wild or in crowded centers. Hygiene isn't just a matter of politeness or comfort, but helps prevent infection and disease and becomes critical in such circumstances.

Wash yourself when possible, paying particular attention to the feet, armpits, crotch, hands, and hair. Those are primary areas for infection and infestation.

If water is scarce, and weather permitting, strip down and expose your body to the air for a little while, without getting sunburned.

Keep Your Hands Clean. This goes even in non-emergency situations. Germs on your hands can infect food and wounds. Wash your hands after handling any material that is likely to carry germs, after visiting the latrine, after caring for the sick, and before handling any food, food utensils, or drinking water. Keep your fingernails closely trimmed and clean.

Keep Your Hair Clean. Your hair can become a haven for bacteria or fleas, lice, and other parasites. Keeping your hair clean, combed, and trimmed helps you avoid this danger.

Keep Your Clothing Clean. Keep your clothing and bedding as clean as possible to reduce the chance of skin infection as well as to decrease the danger of parasitic infestation. Clean your outer clothing whenever it becomes soiled. Wear clean underclothing and socks as much as possible. If water is scarce, clean your clothing by shaking, airing, and sunning it for 2 hours. If you are using a sleeping bag, turn it inside out after each use, fluff it, and air it.

Keep Your Teeth Clean. Thoroughly clean your mouth and teeth with a toothbrush at least once each day. If you don't have a toothbrush, make a chewing stick. Find a twig. Chew one end of the stick to separate the fibers. Now brush your teeth thoroughly. Another is to wrap a clean strip of cloth around your fingers and rub your teeth with it to wipe away food particles. You can also brush your teeth with small amounts of sand, baking soda, salt, or soap. Then rinse your mouth. Flossing your teeth with string or fiber helps oral hygiene.

Take Care of Your Feet. To prevent serious foot problems, break in your shoes before wearing them. Wash and massage your feet daily. Trim your toe-nails straight across. Wear an insole and the proper size of dry socks. Powder and check your feet daily for blisters. If you get a small blister, do not open it. An intact blister is safe from infection. Apply a padding material around the blister to relieve pressure and reduce friction. If the blister bursts, treat it as an open wound. Clean and dress it daily and pad around it.

Keep Camp Site Clean. Do not soil the ground in the camp site area with urine or feces. Use latrines, if available. When latrines are not available, dig "cat holes" and cover the waste. Collect drinking water upstream from the camp site.

Water Procurement

A Mild level stockpile of water was your first task.

What water resources did you list in your Area Study? Which of those are accessible now?

WARNING!
Most Water in Nature is Unsafe to Drink

The spread of Giardia has made most water sources that you used to be able to trust, unsafe. Whatever purification system you use, make sure it will get rid of Giardia. Giardia is spread through animal dropping. If you get this bug, it will seriously degrade you physically and reduce your ability to survive.

By drinking non-potable water you may contract diseases or swallow organisms that can harm you. Examples of such diseases or organisms are—

Dysentery. Severe, prolonged diarrhea with bloody stools, fever, and weakness.

Cholera and typhoid. You may be susceptible to these diseases regardless of inoculations.

Flukes. Stagnant, polluted water—especially in tropical areas—often contains blood flukes. If you swallow flukes, they will bore into the bloodstream, live as parasites, and cause disease.

We have the problem of industrial and chemical pollution almost everywhere. We have little idea what run off is going into the water. Stay away from water that is near roads.

Don't drink downstream of factories that discharge into the water, sewage plants that discharge, mines or, frankly sites of major human habitation.

Don't drink water draining out of utilized farmland.

If you are in an area that has been flooded (aka Katrina), consider all water sources affected by the flooding to be contaminated, even if they were previously considered drinkable.

You have to assume that any water that isn't marked as potable (drinkable) is contaminated. Even in the deepest forest, there is a chance the water is tainted. Always stay on the safe side, because contracting giardia is no fun at all and cholera can be fatal.

WATER SOURCES IN YOUR HOME

We've covered this earlier.

If you have adequate warning, you should fill every available container with potable water. Also fill all tubs and sinks.

There are items in your house that can be used to purify water:

Chlorine Bleach. Standard bleach is 5% chlorine. If the strength is not known go with ten drops per quart or liter for clear water, double that for murky water.

DISINFECTING WATER

Available Chlorine Concentrate	Drops per Quart/Gallon of Clear Water (a drop is 1/8th teaspoon)	Drops per Liter of Clear Water
1.00% to 2.00% Chlorine Concentrate	10 per quart, 40 per gallon	10 per liter
Regular to Ultra Strength 5.25% to 6.00%	2 per quart, 8 per gallon	2 per liter
	Drops per Quart/Gallon of Cloudy Water	Drops per Quart/Gallon of Cloudy Water
1.00% to 2.00% Chlorine Concentrate	20 per quart, 80 per gallon	20 per liter
Regular to Ultra Strength 5.25% to 6.00%	4 per quart, 16 per gallon	4 per liter
Stir the mixture well	Let it stand for 30 minutes	

BOILING WATER

Filter to remove impurities	Use coffee filter, towel, etc.	
Bring to boil	Continue for one minute	
Bring to boil for one minute and	Add 1 minute at boil for every 1,000 feet of altitude	

WATER SOURCES IN NATURE

Warning! Purify any water that you are not positive is drinkable.

Rainwater collected in clean containers is usually safe for drinking. This is the quickest and most effective way to gather potable water.

Lakes, ponds, swamps, springs, streams. Must be purified regardless of how clear and clean it looks. This is especially true if it is anywhere near human settlements.

Underground water: Muddy ground indicates a water supply. You can filter the muddy water or dig down about a foot and gather what collects. It still must be purified.

Snow and ice: Are as pure as the water from which they came, this is particularly true for ice. Do not eat snow or ice without melting first, as doing so will reduce your core body temperature and actually lead to dehydration more than hydration. If you carry a water container in freezing temperatures, remember that it will freeze. Keep your ready source of water inside your coat so remains liquid.

Green bamboo thickets are a source of fresh water. Water from green bamboo is clear and odorless. To get the water, bend a green bamboo stalk, tie it down, and cut off the top. The water will drip freely during the night and collect. Old, cracked bamboo may contain water. Bamboo is a lot more common than you realize. When you did your Area Study, this is something you should have looked for: all the sources of water that you might not have considered before.

Morning dew can provide water. Use an absorbent cloth (this is one case where cotton isn't rotten) or a handful of long grass and wick up moisture that has condensed. You can also tie rags or tufts of fine grass around your ankles and walk through dew-covered grass before sunrise. As the cloth, rags or grass tufts absorb the dew, wring the water into a container. Repeat the process until you have a supply of water or until the dew is gone. This water is consider potable (unless you collect it off of poison ivy or recently fertilized/sprayed grass, etc.)

Banana/plantain trees: Cut down the tree, leaving a stump about a foot high. Scoop out the center, leaving a bowl shaped hollow. Water from the roots will come and being to fill the hollow. The first several fillings will be bitter, but then it was become more palatable. This can supply water for up to four days. If you are going to re-use, cover it to keep insects and bugs out.

Tropical vines: Cut a notch as high as you can reach. Do not drink if it is sticky, milky or bitter-tasting.

Coconuts: The milk from unripe (green) coconuts. The milk from mature coconuts contains a laxative.

Solar water disinfection (SoDis): Given the proliferation of water bottles and the fact you probably have some in your Grab-n-Go bag, car, home, etc. this is a particularly effective method.

Find a clean, clear plastic bottle no more than three liters (1 liter is slightly more than one quart). It needs to be a PET bottle. You can tell by looking on the bottom. Most will say if they are PET or PETE. Otherwise it will have a number. You want a #1. Any other number is a different kind of plastic. The narrower the bottle, the better for solar penetration.

Fill it three quarters full with clear water, or water you have cleaned through sand or whatever tightly woven cloth you have available.

Shake the bottle in order to get as much oxygen as possible into the water.

Fill the rest of the bottle and replace the lid.

Place the bottle in direct sunlight for six to eight hours. You can increase the efficiency by placing the bottle on a reflective surface such as metal or aluminum foil.

If you have to move, hang the bottle on the outside of your pack.

If it isn't sunny out (yeah, you in the Pacific Northwest) or the water is cloudy, leave it in the light for at least two full days. Really, if you live in a cloudy area like the Pacific Northwest get a water filter. In fact, no matter where you live, get a water filter. SODIS is only for extreme situations where there is no other options. Considering you can find empty plastic bottles pretty much anywhere, including the middle of the Pacific Ocean (alas Ancient Mariner, this does not convert salt water), it's a useful one to know.

How SODIS works: The sunlight treats the water through three ways, all involving radiation.

UVA reacts with the oxygen dissolved in the water to produce a highly reactive form with free radicals and hydrogen peroxide, which kills microorganisms.

UVA interferes with the reproductive cycle of bacteria by crippling their DNA.

The sunlight heats the water and once it gets it above 122 degrees F, the disinfection works three times faster.

Like anything else, the combined effect of the three is cumulative. However, this technique DOES NOT remove chemical contamination.

Also, it works better in central latitudes where sunlight is not angled so much. Optimum is 35 degrees latitude north and south.

The plastic bottle should be as new as possible, not colored, and free of scratches. Glass bottles can be used but only as a last resort as they are not as effective.

The thinner the bottle, the better, to allow the sunlight to penetrate.

Of note, SODIS is being used in various places around the world to produce potable water, due to the lack of treated water.

DO NOT DRINK THE FOLLOWING:

Seawater: it is 4 percent salt. It takes 2 quarts of bodily fluids to rid the body of 1 quart of seawater. Thus you are actually dehydrating yourself twice as fast.
Sea Ice: same as seawater.
Blood: Is considered a food, since it's salty, and requires additional bodily fluids to process. It might also transmit disease.
Urine: 2% salt and contains harmful body wastes. There's a reason your body is getting rid of it.
Alcoholic beverages: They dehydrate you and cloud your judgment.

Grab-n-Go bag: You have: Survival straw. Survival filter. Water purification tablets. Use those sparingly if you can find potable water or can purify by other means. You also have at least one water container. Check the instructions on the filters and tablets and use properly.

If the water you find is muddy, stagnant, and/or foul smelling, you can clear the water by placing it in a container and letting it stand for 12 hours. Or by passing it through cloth multiple times. Or through sand. But these procedures only clear the water and make it more palatable. You will still have to purify it.

To purify water the rule is to boil it for one minute at sea level.
Add one minute for each thousand feet above sea level.

Some rules of thumb if things are extreme and you must drink without time or ability to purify:

Running water is better than still water.

Water coming out of a spring is better than running water.

Clear water is usually better than cloudy or discolored water (but only in an emergency as you can't see what will make you sick).

Avoid water that has algae in it.

Avoid swamp or marshland water.

Scavenge

Full, unopened, water bottles are everywhere in our civilization. Don't just check stores. Homes. Businesses. Vending machines. Inside cars and trucks. More under the section on Scavenge.

In an extreme survival system when you have gone into Scavenge mode, find an abandoned house that has a water system. Find the filters for the purification system. In my current house, my kitchen sink has a two filter system that could be cannibalized and used. The key is that it requires pressure to push water through the system. But gravity provides pressure, slowly but surely.

Sustain

Look around. Listen. Smell. Watch animals. They need water.

Make sure you clearly mark and separate potable from non-potable water containers. Never, ever, mix the two.

A source of drinking water should be your priority in finding a BOHS. There are easily defendable locales such as an island or a prison, but do they have water?

Food Procurement

Food is not an issue for mild emergencies. We can survive a while without food. Since you have your supplies in your house and your Grab-n-Go bags ready, you are able to live off your stockpile.

Your baseline in your house is a 3 days non-perishable supply. The same for your Grab-n-Go bag. That gives you six days. There is also food in your car.

And initially, on top of that, you have your everyday pantry and refrigerator.

As we move from mild into moderate emergencies, and the time gets longer, food will start to become more of an issue.

Mod/Ex Food

You need an adequate amount of food to stay healthy. Without food your mental and physical capabilities will deteriorate rapidly, and you will become weak. Food replenishes the substances that your body uses and provides energy. Food provides vitamins, minerals, salts, and other elements essential to good health.

The two basic sources of food are plants and animals (including fish). In varying degrees both provide the calories, carbohydrates, fats, and proteins needed for normal daily body functions.

Calories are a measure of heat and potential energy. The average person needs roughly 2,000 calories per day to function at a minimum level. In extreme situations we can go down to 800 calories but not for long. I recommend 2,400 calories as your planning baseline.

Plant Foods:

These foods provide carbohydrates—the main source of energy. Many plants provide enough protein to keep the body at normal efficiency. Although plants may not provide a balanced diet, they will sustain you even in the arctic, where meat's heat-producing qualities are normally essential. Many plant foods such as nuts and seeds will give you enough protein and oils for normal efficiency. Roots, green vegetables, and plant food containing natural sugar will provide calories and carbohydrates that give the body natural energy.

The food value of plants becomes more and more important if you are eluding the enemy or if you are in an area where wildlife is scarce.

You can dry plants by wind, air, sun, or fire. This retards spoilage so that you can store or carry the plant food with you to use when needed.

You can obtain plants more easily and more quietly than meat.

Animal Foods:

To get meat, you need to know the habits of, and how to capture/kill various wildlife.

To satisfy your immediate food needs, first seek the more abundant and more easily obtained wildlife, such as insects, crustaceans, mollusks, fish, and reptiles.

Disclaimer: If you want to learn how hunt, trap, fish, skin animals, butcher them, etc. *after* an emergency or disaster happens is not the best time. The smarter plan is to have someone on your survival team who knows how to do this or learn to do it beforehand. I will give some basics from which you can expand.

Food is an area where people will go into scavenge mode and, if resourceful, can stay there for a long time. Long enough, most importantly, to begin planting crops. If civilization collapses, we will follow the historical path our ancestors did in building back up: after scavenging no longer works, those who are still alive, will become hunter/gatherers, while some will move right to farming. The danger with farming is that it makes you stationery, which makes you a target for scavengers.

It's a vicious formula.

The same with having domesticated animals. Great idea, and they are moveable, but they are also targets.

For Your Home

Once you go through your food stockpile, what is left? Don't assume some food is inedible just because its past the expiration date. Expiration dates were covered in Prepare under Food.

Grow a garden.

Plant the seeds at the appropriate time. This is a sustainable source of food. It is seasonal in most places, unless you have a greenhouse. However, it is also a fixed location. Also, consider the fact that you will target gardens that have been abandoned during the scavenging phase, so you should have a basic familiarity with some of the staple foods that are usually grown.

Unless you're an expert gardener, stick to some basics if you are going to be in one area for a while and need sustainability. Remember, you can hide a garden among wild growth, but that it also will be food for animals.

Beans: Green Beans grow fast and replenish. Normally planted in early summer. Many varieties need poles or branches to grow on. They are good sources of fiber, calcium and Vitamins A, C and K.

Peas: Very easy to grow. Fast growing. Source of fiber, protein, and several vitamins.

Peppers: Plant after last frost. High in Vitamins A and C.

Potatoes: Plant a month after last frost. High in fiber and Vitamin A and C.

Lettuce: Easy to grow.

Cucumbers: Warm weather crop. Easy to grow. Pick constantly and it will continue to yield results. Vitamins A, C, K and potassium.

Tomatoes: Plant in late spring and/or later summer. Vitamins A, C, E, K, potassium, thiamine and Niacin.

This is an over-view. As with many specialties, there are two factors that need to be considered during your scavenging phase before you go to sustainment and needing to grow food:

Find people who know how to grow food to be part of your team.

Scavenge books on how to garden, material and tools for gardening, locate hidden sites to plant food, and make seed scavenging a higher priority as the sustainment phase comes closer.

Food In Nature
Depending on your skills, your location and your needs, you might turn to food in nature before you turn to scavenging. We'll tackle some basic techniques here.

Gathering: cultivated plants, wild edible plants, insects, birds eggs.

Think of two types of edible plants. Cultivated crops and certain plants in the wild.

When you did your Area Study, you noted what crops are grown in your locale. Which are edible? How do you make them edible? Some, such as corn, as obvious. Others require more study.

Edible plants have such a wide array across so many different climates and environs, there isn't the space to cover them here. Particularly to describe them.

A person who can recognize plants, which are edible, which are useful for other purposes such as herbs, and also grow them, is as valuable to a survival team than a top notch hunter.

Hunting

You need the means to hunt. Normally that means firearms, although skilled crossbow and bow hunters will be very valuable. Firearms have a noise signature. Arrows don't.

As far as field expedient weapons such as spears, bows, etc. that is beyond our scope here. Not only do you have to make them, you'd have to become proficient. The time and energy put into such field-expedient weapons is almost prohibitive except in the most extreme survival situations.

Hunting is recommended for large game, with a large return in terms of not only meat but other by-products.

If you have a .22 caliber rifle, the sound signature is much less, and you can carry many more rounds. But you will also be hunting much smaller game. Remember, though, that there is more small game than large game.

All mammals are edible and excellent protein sources (except the polar bear and bearded seal which have toxins in their livers). Remember, though, that a wounded animal, even something as small as a raccoon, can cause nasty wounds which run the risk of infection.

Unless you are already a hunter, focus on . . .

Trapping: In your Grab-n-Go bag are ready made snares. Remember? Here they are in case you skipped the Prepare book:
Versatile Snares: https://amzn.to/2BN29rG

You might have wondered at the time why they were included. Now you know. While there are field expedient traps you can make, this is the simplest and most effective way.

Snares are very effective for harvesting small game. They were used by our ancient ancestors and they still work. The ones you have are lightweight, easy to pack and relatively easy to use.

Your snare is made from tightly wound steel cable five or more feet long. It has a one way locking mechanism on one end and a swivel and loop on the other.

First, find a trail where the game you're after is known to travel. Look for worn trails through the underbrush.

Anchor your snare. Use wire, such as from a coat hanger, slide it through the loop, and tie it around the base of a tree or post. Make sure the wire can't be pulled apart or unwound by the animal as it fights the trap.

Find a stick as the stand for the snare. Prop it up between the anchor point and the loop for snare. Have the slide lock of the loop about a half inch in front of the support. Essentially you're hanging a noose down over the trail. Once you're in place, push the stick down into the ground fixing it in place. The loop must be at the proper height for your target—where it's head would go into the loop. This is from 3 inches to 10 inches off the ground.

Set multiple snares to increase your odds. This is another way trapping is more effective than hunting.

Check your traps every day. The animal will be dead because the sliding lock closes around their necks and either cuts off circulation or breaks their neck during their initial struggle to get free.

Some notes on trapping:

Animals have to drink. Trails to watering holes are excellent places to emplace snares.

Don't disturb the area where you emplace your snare any more than necessary. Have all your parts ready, then go to the location and emplace. Do not use freshly cut vegetation in either the snare or to channel animals as the sap gives off an odor. Most mammals you are hunting depend heavily on their sense of smell for protection. You can use the fluid from the gall and urine bladders of previous kills to mask your scent. Coat your hands with it before assembling the snare.

You can build a channel along the trail to ensure the target runs into the snare, but odds are doing so will leave too much odor and visual sign. However, few wild animals will back up.

You can bait a trap, but it must be a bait the target wants and isn't readily available all around. Peanut butter is a good bait. So is salt.

Fishing

In your Grab-n-Go bag, you have some basic fishing essentials. Line, hooks. What is your experience level?

Some basic guidelines on survival fishing:

Fish tend to feed before a storm, not after.

Light attracts fish at night.

Fish gather where there are deep pools, overhanging trees and brush, and around submerged foliage and logs that offer shelter.

There are no poisonous freshwater fish. Catfish do have needle-like protrusions on their dorsal fins that can inflict painful wounds, which leave you open to infection.

Cook all freshwater fish to kill parasites.

Cook saltwater fish caught inside of a reef or under the influence of a freshwater source. Fish caught in the open sea can be eaten raw because of the salt water. However, there are some poisonous saltwater fish such as porcupine, triggerfish, cowfish, oilfish, thorn fish and red snapper.

How to fish:

Identify the best location.

Set multiple lines. Use trees branches hanging over the water instead of poles. Tie a baited hook, with a weight, on a line. For bait use live worms. Pretty much anything that crawls and you can put on the hook will serve. Once you start catching fish, use can use pieces of those fish as bait.

Scavenge

Reverse the food distribution network. The consumer gets food from a store. A store gets food delivered from a warehouse or a local producer. The warehouse gets food from where? Locally? Another distribution center? This goes on until we get to the true source of the food.

Where in that chain can you intervene and get food?

More on this under Scavenge, as food is just one many items you will be looking for.

Sustain

Grow a garden. If you have the ground, plant the seeds at the appropriate time. This is a sustainable source of food. It is seasonal in most places, unless you have a greenhouse. However, it is also a fixed location.

Be a hunter/gather on the move.

Barter: Some skills will be worth others paying for in terms of food. Medical expertise is one such skill set.

Building a Shelter and Starting a Fire

Your home is your primary shelter. You've also designated a NOHS.

Beyond that, unless you're in the middle of nowhere, mankind has built millions of possible shelters, ranging from homes, factories, schools, churches, warehouses, etc.

If none of these work, your Grab-n-Go bag has shelter, ranging from a tent, to a poncho, to an emergency sleeping bag.

A shelter is anything that can protect against not only the elements, but also danger. That means other people, but also the danger attendant with various emergencies and catastrophes.

In extreme emergencies, shelter can become the number one priority not only because we can survive only 3 hours with an un-regulated body temperature, but also because shelter can protect us against various other threats. So let's start with . . .

EMERGENCY SHELTERS

A field expedient shelter out in nature takes several times longer to build than you think. Consider that in terms of the threat.

Location is the first consideration. If there isn't a man-made scavenge-able one available, is there a natural shelter? Tree well, where a tree has fallen and the roots have opened a large hole? Burned out log? Cave? Rock overhang? A log with a dry spot underneath?

You face a key decision if you are losing body temperature. Do you build the shelter first or the fire? If it's raining and you know you can't get a fire going, then the shelter comes first. If the warmth of exertion from building the shelter won't stop the onset of hypothermia, then the fire first.

A tarp shelter is the most basic shelter. Using the poncho and paracord that should be in all your Grab-n-Go bags, or scavenged from your environment.

A few keys apply when putting one together:

Look for natural or manmade surroundings that give you a good location and enhance the shelter. Incorporating a wall, a blown down tree, a large rock, etc. as part of the shelter is a good idea. Notice prevailing wind. Have your opening facing away.

One key to all emergency shelters: Smaller is better! First, a smaller shelter is easier to build, using less materials. Second, it will keep your body heat enclosed. Third, it is less noticeable.

There are five main areas to consider for an emergency shelter:

Urban: The most important aspect to consider here is other human beings. In an extreme emergency, survival is more important than etiquette and sometimes even law. When I lived in South Korea, when the alert siren went off, everyone was required to go indoors via the closest door to you. Didn't matter whose it was. They had to let you in. During a civil disturbance or a riot or extreme emergency, don't hesitate to knock on doors, whether it be homes or shops, to get out of danger.

There are hazards to watch out for besides unfriendly people such as downed power lines, broken water mains and unstable ruins.

Cities are three dimensional. Look up. Going to upper floors of buildings gives you the high ground and a more easily defended position. However, it also traps you. Cities have a veritable maze underneath them. Subway lines, sewers, communication tunnels, steam tunnels. No human being knows the exact extent of what is under New York City. Chicago has old coal tunnels that few people are aware of. These are things you looked for in your Area Study.

A key to remember with all emergency shelter in crowded areas is that others will also be seeking shelter.

Forest: The most desperate shelter is the debris hut. Just gather as much material around you as you can and bury yourself in it. If you have any sort of waterproof material put it as the outer layer, just like with clothing. Putting waterproof material next to your body traps your body's moisture and makes you wet.

Use as many branches and sticks to make a solid frame. Tie some together, or lacking paracord or other tying material, jam them into the ground and against each other. Then layer branches, leaves, sod, etcetera over the framework as tightly as possible without collapsing it.

Jungle: Essential the same as the debris hut, except you have more material to work with. You have vines, hollow shoots, larger leaves and the ground is usually softer and often provides clay. A key in the jungle shelter is get out of the moisture. In a swamp you want to put your shelter on the highest piece of ground you can find. Even a few inches can make a difference.

Snow/Winter: While survival shows have people building igloos and snow caves, these are time and labor intensive. Certainly, if you have both resources and time you can build them. However, my experience is that a snow trench is the simplest to build, if you have a poncho or other material to cover it. Once more, smaller is better. Dig a trench long enough and narrow enough for you to get into. Deep enough for you to be below the top surface of the snow. Make sure you put something at the bottom to keep your body off the snow. Put the poncho or tarp over the top, using snow to anchor each side. Leave a small opening you can slide in and out of and that you can fix in place.

A snow cave is similar except you are going further into the snow (thus requiring deeper snow) and leaving a snow roof in place. To fix the sides of a trench or cave, and the roof of a cave, use a candle or lighter to glaze the snow, briefly melting it, then allowing the temperature to turn it into ice.

Desert: Are you going to be traveling or not? If you're going to be moving you need a shelter for the day, to keep you as cool as possible and out of the sun, as you'll be traveling at night. If you're not traveling, then your shelter also has to work at night. As we noted discussing desert survival, it often gets quite cold at night in the desert.

Use any vegetation available such as a juniper tree or sagebrush. Use piled up sand or rocks for one side of a shelter. If you can, dig into the ground. A belowground shelter can reduce the temperature thirty degrees.

BUILDING A FIRE

You have windproof lighters and matches in your Grab-n-Go bags and on your survival vest. Also a magnesium fire starter which you've practiced with.

Some caveats on fire starting. Make sure whatever you start doesn't get out of control. Fire is our friend until it becomes our enemy.

There are keys to starting any fire. First is gathering the proper flammables. They should be dry. If your environment is damp or wet, search for dry material under hanging rocks, under logs, or even gather damp material and put inside your shirt to use your body warmth to dry it out. Breaking damp sticks should expose a dry portion. Don't use soggy or rotten wood.

You need three piles:

Tinder: Dry, flammable material that needs only a few sparks to ignite. Thin, fibrous plant material. Fine steel wool. Tinder is easy to ignite but does not sustain fire. So you need . . .

Kindling: Slightly larger organic material that feeds the fire initially. Dry wood chips, twigs, dry strips of bark, dry grass stalks, refuse such as paper.

Firewood: Thicker branches and logs take longer to ignite, but once they do, they sustain the fire longer.

Field expedient ways:

Hand drill: The easiest field expedient way to build a fire is also the most labor intensive. Use a piece of hardwood as the fireboard. Make a notch in it with a knife or pointed rock. You need a two-foot-long stick whose tip fits into the notch. Surround the notch with tinder. Roll the stick between your palms (wear gloves if you have them), causing friction. Enough friction causes heat. It will start smoking and ignite the kindling. Slowly add kindling to build the fire

Mirror/Glass: This requires two items. Sunlight and a parabolic mirror or lens. The reflector of a flashlight, the clean inside of a soda can are possibilities in a pinch. A clear bottle filled with water. Anything that can focus the rays of the sun.

Sustaining a long term fire: keep the flames going. If a fire burns down to embers, you use the core of that to restart the fire, using the same flow as starting a new fire: tinder, kindling, firewood. Tossing firewood on embers could disperse the embers and cause you to start over again.

Navigating and Tracking

In an emergency situation, especially moderate to extreme, it is highly possible you will have to move from point A to point B. It is likely you won't have a GPS to do that with.

So let's walk through basic land navigation before briefly touching on tracking and evasion.

Based on your preparation, you've already downloaded or purchased topographic maps.

Your map is a very valuable document. Treat is as one. Keep it in the waterproof map case you have and keep it tied off to your body.

When you look at a topo map, you immediately see that it's different than your road map. Features on it include:

Roads, buildings, boundaries, railways, power transmission lines and more.

Water: lakes, rivers, streams, swamps, rapids, kraken, etc.

Relief: mountains, valleys, slopes, depressions, ridges, knolls, gnomes, etc.

Vegetation: forested or clear areas, orchards, vineyards, Ents, etc.

Toponymy: a fancy word for the names of the various things on the map.

Use the map legend to learn how to use the symbols, colors and lines on the map.

Scale is the relationship between size on the map and in the real world. One thing I've noted on many GPS systems is that they don't indicate scale since they give directions and distance. This can be disorienting. Everything always looks a lot closer on a map than when you're walking.

Legend

It gives you a guide to the various symbols on the map. The types of roads will be defined in the Legend.

Contour lines

These designate elevation. If you trace a contour line on the map, you are tracing a line of equal elevation. If you walked that line, you will not go up or down. Check the legend for the contour interval—this is critical. There's a big difference between a 10 meter contour interval and a 50 meter one. As you go from one contour line to the next, that is the contour interval difference. Usually contour interval is based on the terrain the map covers. Relatively flat terrain will have very short interval, while mountainous terrain might have intervals as great as 100 meters. Every fifth contour line is an index and labeled with a number.

The closer lines are, the steeper the terrain. When they're piled on top of each other, that means a cliff. Do not walk off it. If they are very far apart, that equals relatively smooth terrain. Notice how contour lines always dive in toward streams and rivers.

The key to using a map is orienting it to the terrain. While there are many field-expedient ways of doing this, the easiest is to orient using a compass. Next easiest is to use roads or easily identifiable terrain features around you.

But suppose you don't have a compass or readily identifiable terrain features?

Using the sun

The sun rises in the east and sets in the west. Depending on time of year and where you in terms of latitude, that will shift north and south in degrees. In the northern hemisphere, the sun will be due south when at its highest point in the sky, or when an object casts no appreciable shadow. In the southern hemisphere, this same noon day sun will mark due north. In the northern hemisphere, shadows will move clockwise. Shadows will move counterclockwise in the southern hemisphere.

The shadow methods used for direction finding are the shadow-tip and watch methods.

Shadow-Tip Method

Find a straight stick 3 feet long and an open, level spot on which the stick will cast a definite shadow.

Step 1. Place the stick or branch into the ground where it will cast a distinctive shadow. Mark the shadow's tip. This first shadow mark is always west —**everywhere** on earth.

Step 2. Wait until the shadow tip moves a few inches. Mark the shadow tip's new position.

Step 3. Draw a straight line through the two marks to obtain an approximate east-west line.

Step 4. Stand with the first mark (west) to your left and the second mark to your right-you are now facing north. This fact is true **everywhere** on earth.

The Watch Method

You can also determine direction using a common or analog watch—one that has hands. The direction will be accurate if you are using true local time, without any changes for daylight savings time. Remember, the further you are from the equator, the more accurate this method will be. If you only have a digital watch, you can overcome this obstacle. Quickly draw a watch on a circle of paper with the correct time on it and use it to determine your direction at that time.

In the northern hemisphere, hold the watch horizontal and point the hour hand at the sun. Bisect the angle between the hour hand and the 12 o'clock mark to get the north-south line. If there is any doubt as to which end of the line is north, remember that the sun rises in the east, sets in the west, and is due south at noon. The sun is in the east before noon and in the west after noon.

Note: If your watch is set on daylight savings time, use the midway point between the hour hand and 1 o'clock to determine the north-south line.

In the southern hemisphere, point the watch's 12 o'clock mark toward the sun and a midpoint halfway between 12 and the hour hand will give you the north-south line.

Using the Stars

Your location in the Northern or Southern Hemisphere determines which constellation you use to determine your north or south direction.

The Northern Sky

The main constellations to learn are the Ursa Major, also known as the Big Dipper or the Plow, and Cassiopeia. Neither of these constellations ever set. They are always visible on a clear night. Use them to locate Polaris, also known as the polestar or the North Star. The North Star forms part of the Little Dipper handle and can be confused with the Big Dipper. Prevent confusion by using both the Big Dipper and Cassiopeia together. The Big Dipper and Cassiopeia are always directly opposite each other and rotate counterclockwise around Polaris, with Polaris in the center. The Big Dipper is a seven star constellation in the shape of a dipper. The two stars forming the outer lip of this dipper are the "pointer stars" because they point to the North Star. Mentally draw a line from the outer bottom star to the outer top star of the Big Dipper's bucket. Extend this line about five times the distance between the pointer stars. You will find the North Star along this line.

Cassiopeia has five stars that form a shape like a "W" on its side. The North Star is straight out from Cassiopeia's center star. After locating the North Star, locate the North Pole or true north by drawing an imaginary line directly to the earth.

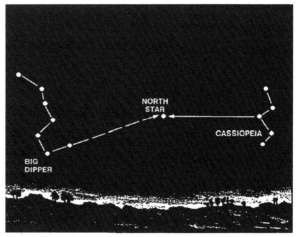

Figure 18-3. The Big Dipper and Cassiopeia.

The Southern Sky

Because there is no star bright enough to be easily recognized near the south celestial pole, a constellation known as the Southern Cross is used as a sign post to the South (Figure18-4).

The Southern Cross or Crux has five stars. Its four brightest stars form a cross that tilts to one side. The two stars that make up the cross's long axis are the pointer stars. To determine south, imagine a distance five times the distance between. These stars and the point where this imaginary line ends is in the general direction of south. Look down to the horizon from this imaginary point and select a landmark to steer by. In a static survival situation you can fix this location in daylight if you drive stakes in the ground at night to point the way.

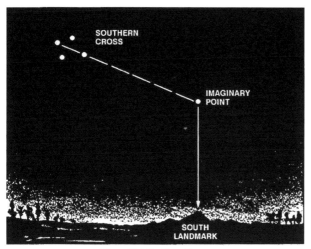

Figure 18-4. Southern Cross.

Navigation.

Water flows downhill. That sounds basic, but sometimes we need to remind ourselves of the basics.

Study a map of your region. What are the major streams and rivers? Where do they join? How many bridges cross them? Where? Remember, bridges are chokepoints.

Are there any significant terrain features in your area that are noticeable from a distance? Pilots Peak in Utah was a landmark for many people traveling west.

Know your pace count. This is how many times your right foot hits the ground per one hundred meters. This allows you to stay oriented. You can go to the local high school and pace off one hundred yards, which is close to one hundred meters (a yard is slightly longer). But remember, that will be on flat ground. Pace count changes greatly when you move through rough terrain and are carrying a backpack.

Tracking and Evasion

This usually comes into play during an extreme emergency when there is conflict among people. In order to understand how to evade being tracked down, you need to first understand how to track someone.

The real key to tracking someone is not examining bent twigs, or marks in the dirt, but rather understanding the mindset and habits of whatever you are tracking. Predators tend to cluster near water sources in areas where water is scarce. Rather than tracking down their prey, they let their prey come to them. People tend to take the easiest path. That's why ambushes are set up along paths and choke points.

Where will whoever or whatever you are tracking be going? What is their destination? If you're very sure of their destination, perhaps you can get there before them. Will they need food? Water? When setting your snares for food, this is a key consideration.

To evade someone tracking you, you must avoid the easy way. You must break bad habits. You must confuse them. You must make it difficult for them to follow.

My first platoon sergeant told me an interesting thing: few people ever look up. Remember in *Hunger Games* when the heroine hides up in a tree? Like everything else, this is a double-edged thing: you might not be noticed, but if you are, as she was, you are trapped.

One of the best ways to avoid being followed is to use water. Few people want to wade through water or go into that swamp. A little discomfort can be worth your life.

Here are keys to evasion:

If ever captured, try to escape quickly. The longer you remain a prisoner, the lower your chances of escape.

If ever arrested, say nothing. You have the right to remain silent, so remain silent.

Don't be noticeable. Ever watch a crowd? Ever see the people who stand out? You don't want to be that person. A rule of survival on the New York subway is to not make eye contact. One of my rules is to never poke the crazy person. When walking down the street, avoid eye contact and all contact with those who could possibly be threats. When avoiding a riot or civil unrest, the same applies.

If your team has to evade, you must make an important decision: whether to break the group up into pairs or try to evade as a team. Remember, of course, that you are evading to a point, usually your ERP. So if any team members are captured, you must assume they will give up the location of the ERP. On the other hand, pairs have a greater chance of evasion than a large group.

Don't leave tracks. This seems obvious, but few of us have ever thought about it. And even fewer have ever looked behind ourselves to see if we are leaving tracks.

In Conclusion

The odds that you will have to track or evade are low in a mild or moderate emergency. But the odds you will have to land navigate without electronic aid isn't so low. Make sure you have maps, both road and topographical. Make sure you have a basic understanding of the terrain around you. Practice your routes from your home to you IRP and ERP and on to the Hide Site.

When traveling, plan your route and plan alternate routes.

Specific Environments

Since you've done your Area Study, you have a good idea of what you are facing in your area of operations.

Depending on where you live or travel, you must make special arrangements for extremes in terrain and weather. I'm going to briefly cover key points in preparing for four special environments: cold weather, desert, tropical and water survival.

The climate of the United States varies due to differences in latitude, and a range of geographic features, including mountains and deserts. West of the 100th meridian, roughly a line along the border of Kansas and Colorado and going up and down, much of the US is semi-arid to arid. This includes desert in the Southwest. East of that line, the climate is humid continental in the north, humid temperate in the central and mid-Atlantic and humid subtropical in the Gulf and southern Atlantic areas. The southern tip of Florida is tropical. In higher elevations in the western mountains the climate is alpine. Alaska is largely subarctic. Hawaii is tropical.

Let's cover key points about four basic environments

COLD WEATHER

I commanded an A-Team in the 10th Special Forces Group (Airborne). 10th Group had the distinction of being the 'cold weather' Group, since it was oriented toward high altitude environments. We often sent teams to Finland, Norway, Denmark and other cold regions for training. An annual event was Winter Warfare Training, where each battalion deployed for almost two months. We learned to ski, then survive and operate in high altitude and cold weather. My first winter warfare was an eye-opening experience for me. There were many tricks of the trade learned, but several key lessons:

1) Everything takes at least twice as long to achieve in cold weather.

2) Fire is eventually an essential. Whether for melting snow and ice into water, cooking meals, drying out clothing and gear, or warming people up.

3) Moving on snow with equipment is extraordinarily hard.

4) Cold weather affects equipment in different ways. One key to remember is that any exposed water container will freeze. We quickly learned to keep our water container inside our clothing, allowing our body to keep it from freezing. The same with thawing out our next meal.

The key, like everything else, is to be properly prepared at all times. Not just at home, but especially when traveling in your car. Also, at work.

There are two types of cold weather environments: wet or dry. New England, for example, is wet cold. The Rocky Mountains are dry cold. We took more cold weather casualties when we trained in the Adirondacks at a lower elevation than when we trained in Utah at high altitude based on the difference between wet cold and dry cold.

When we conducted a security test of the Alaskan pipeline in November, we ran into wet cold conditions. I ended up having to medevac one of my weapons sergeants because he'd been a previous cold weather casualty and walking through the Alaskan tundra (frozen at night, thawing in the day) took him down. This is something else to consider with team members: who has had previous cold or hot weather injuries.

Wind chill is the effect of moving air on exposed flesh. Wind always exacerbates the situation, which is why your outer garment should not only be water resistant, but wind resistant. A key in building shelter is to get out of the wind. Wind multiplies the effect of low temperatures.

Even when there is no wind, you will create the equivalent wind by skiing, running, being towed on skis behind a vehicle, working around aircraft that produce wind. One of my coldest experiences where I almost suffered instant frostbite was loading an injured soldier on board a Blackhawk helicopter at altitude in a cold environment. I made the mistake of briefly taking my gloves off and almost paid for it.

Always keep your head covered. Because there is much blood circulation in the head, most of which is on the surface, you can lose heat quickly if you do not cover your head. This is also why scalp wounds tend to bleed profusely.

There are four basic principles to follow to keep warm. An easy way to remember these basic principles is to use the word COLD—

C keep clothing *Clean.*

O avoid *Overheating. (once more: sweating is very dangerous in the cold)*

L wear clothes *Loose* and in *Layers.*

D keep clothing *Dry.*

C Keep clothing clean. This principle is always important for sanitation and comfort. In winter, it is also important from the standpoint of warmth. Clothes matted with dirt and grease lose much of their insulation value. Heat can escape more easily from the body through the clothing's crushed or filled up air pockets.

O Avoid overheating. When you get too hot, you sweat and your clothing absorbs the moisture. This affects your warmth in two ways: dampness decreases the insulation quality of clothing, and as sweat evaporates, your body cools. Adjust your clothing so that you do not sweat. Do this by partially opening your parka or jacket, by removing an inner layer of clothing, by removing heavy outer mittens, or by throwing back your parka hood or changing to lighter headgear. The head and hands act as efficient heat dissipaters when overheated.

L Wear your clothing loose and in layers. Wearing tight clothing and footgear restricts blood circulation and invites cold injury. It also decreases the volume of air trapped between the layers, reducing its insulating value. Several layers of lightweight clothing are better than one equally thick layer of clothing, because the layers have dead-air space between them. The dead-air space provides extra insulation. Also, layers of clothing allow you to take off or add clothing layers to prevent excessive sweating or to increase warmth.

D Keep clothing dry. In cold temperatures, your inner layers of clothing can become wet from sweat and your outer layer, if not water repellent, can become wet from snow and frost melted by body heat. Wear water repellent outer clothing, if available. It will shed most of the water collected from melting snow and frost. Before entering a heated shelter, brush off the snow and frost. Despite the precautions you take, there will be times when you cannot keep from getting wet. At such times, drying your clothing may become a major problem. On the march, hang your damp mittens and socks on your rucksack. In freezing temperatures, the wind and sun will dry this clothing. You can also place damp socks or mittens, unfolded, near your body so that your body heat can dry them. In a campsite, hang damp clothing inside the shelter near the top, using drying lines or improvised racks. Dry leather items slowly. If no other means are available for drying your boots, put them between your sleeping bag shell and liner. Your body heat will help to dry the leather.

A heavy, down-lined sleeping bag is a valuable piece of survival gear in cold weather. Ensure the down remains dry. If wet, it loses a lot of its insulation value. If you do not have a sleeping bag, you can make one out of parachute cloth or similar material and natural dry material, such as leaves, pine needles, or moss. Place the dry material between two layers of the material. This is a field expedient piece of equipment sewn together by the survivors of the plane crash in the Andes that helped save their lives.

Dehydration

When bundled up in many layers of clothing during cold weather, you may be unaware that you are losing body moisture. Your heavy clothing absorbs the moisture that normally evaporates in the air. You must drink water to replace this loss of fluid. Your need for water is as great in a cold environment as it is in a warm environment even though you don't feel as thirsty. In fact, we often don't want to drink water when we're cold.

One way to tell if you are becoming dehydrated is to check the color of your urine on snow. If your urine makes the snow dark yellow, you are becoming dehydrated and you need to replace body fluids. If it makes the snow light yellow to no color, your body fluids have a more normal balance. You can also smell the sharp odor of the urine when someone is dehydrated. It's very hard to make people drink water in a cold environment, which makes dehydration a particular danger. A team leader must keep track to make sure every person stays hydrated.

DESERT

A large swatch of our country is either desert or high desert. There was a reason the early wagon trains going west dreaded crossing the desert as much as they did getting through the mountains.

Low rainfall is the most obvious environmental factor in an arid area. A desert is general classified as an area that received less than ten inches of rain in a year. For example, Phoenix receives slightly over eight inches a year on average.

Intense sunlight and heat are present in all arid areas. Air temperature can go well over 100 degrees F every day. The highest recorded temperature in the United States was 134 F in Death Valley. Heat comes from more than direct sunlight. Hot wind, reflective heat (sun bouncing off the sand/ground/rocks) and conductive heat when you make direct contact with the ground.

The ground is going to be much hotter than the air. For example, if the air is 110 F, the ground could easily be 140 F.

Your requirements for water will be much higher in a desert environment. Shelter is as critical in this environment as in a cold weather environment. If you have to move, travel at night to avoid the sun. Equipment behaves differently under extreme temperatures. High temperatures affect batteries adversely and they will not last as long as usual.

Wide Temperature Range: Temperatures will vary widely in desert areas, particularly high desert. During the day it can be well over 100 F and at night quickly drop to below 50 F. This means you have to be prepared for both extremes, especially with clothing.

Sparse Vegetation: There is little vegetation in a desert area. This means you'll have a tougher time making an expedient shelter. The best shelter you can find during the day is in the shadows. The temperature in a shaded area is significantly less than in the open. Also, reflective and conductive heat will be much less.

A problem in the desert is estimating distance. On average, we underestimate distance by a factor of three. What looks like a mile away, is actually three miles away.

Water requirements: Your body sheds heat by sweating. The hotter you are, the more you sweat. While in a cold weather environment you can modulate this by shedding layers of clothing, in a desert you don't have this option. What you can do is conserve your sweat as much as possible. Wear clothing that covers you. This not only protects you from the sun and the wind heat, but it absorbs your sweat and keeps it next to your body as long as possible rather than getting immediately evaporated.

Limit eating as much as possible. Food requires water for digestion, so you are walking a fine line. Remember that water is more vital than food.

You cannot trust your sense of thirst to determine your water requirement. It's been found that a person who relies on thirst drinks only two-thirds of what they actually require.

TROPICAL

A tropical region has high temperatures, heavy rainfall, and high humidity. Tropics cover about seven percent of the world's land surface but contain over fifty percent of the species. Temperatures rarely fall before freezing, unless one is at altitude.

Since the tropics are near the equator, day and night are usually of roughly equal length. Night tends to come quickly, as does dawn.

On the plus side, the tropical environment provides plenty of raw material for shelter, food and water is plentiful. On the negative side, germs and parasites multiply at an alarming rate.

WATER

When we think of water survival, our minds turn to the ocean. However, the worst maritime disaster in United States history, with more loss of life than the *Titanic*, occurred on the Mississippi River when the *Sultana* exploded, caught on fire, and sank.

Even in a desert environment, water can cause an emergency in terms of flash floods which will be covered shortly.

Water covers seventy-five percent of the earth's surface. Seventy percent of that is oceans and seas. When I lived on Whidbey Island, I was on a ferry several times a week. Even though it was a short ride, it still had the possibility of an emergency occurring.

The first priority to prepare for a water emergency is to know how to swim. Sounds basic, but many people don't know how to swim. It's never too late to take a course in basic survival swimming.

If stranded on the open ocean, you face numerous hazards. Waves, wind, extreme heat or cold, the sun, are just a few. Shelter depends on how you're stranded. Shelter, water and food are the priorities.

Any time you are on board a ship or boat make sure you know where the survival gear is. Where are the lifeboats? The life preservers? What supplies are in the lifeboats? How many does each carry? Make sure you know your route to your evacuation point.

If you are in an aircraft and survive a water landing, get clear of the aircraft as quickly as possible and in an upwind direction. Stay clear of fuel-covered water. Try to find other survivors.

When you get that briefing about a water landing at the start of a flight, one thing they sometimes mention but is often not noted is that you do not inflate your life vest until you are outside of the aircraft. If you inflate inside and the aircraft begins to flood, you could be trapped inside by the buoyancy.

Your best protection against the effects of cold water is to get out of the water as quickly as possible, whether it be a life raft or a piece of wreckage. Stay dry, and insulate your body from the cold surface of the bottom of the raft. If in the water keep your head and neck out of the water. Wearing life preservers increases the predicted survival time as body position in the water increases the chance of survival.

Specific Man-Made Threats

CAR

We covered what to have in your car, but here are specific situations where you should know what to do before they occur.

Tornados. If you can see a tornado, drive away from it as quickly and safely as possible. Move at right angles to the tornado. To get an idea of the path of the storm, pick a stationary object near you and watch how the tornado moves in relation to that object. If it is moving to your left, drive to the right and vice versa. If it doesn't seem to be moving left or right, then it's either coming right at you or away from you. If it's getting bigger, guess which of the two? Get out of the car and seek safety in a building or culvert if you have the time.

If you can, stop and seek shelter in a building or underground, such as a culvert. If you get caught while in the car, do NOT get out of the car. It's not safe, but it's better than the options. Pull off the road, out of traffic, because that other idiot is still going to be barreling down the road at 70 miles an hour even though he can't see. Make sure you have your set belt on. Put your head down to avoid broken glass and hurled objects. Cover your head with a blanket or jacket. Do NOT seek shelter under overpasses. Tornados can move at sixty miles an hour, so think hard before trying to out-run one.

Fire: 33 cars catch on fire every hour and 18% of all fires occur on roads. So it's not as rare as you think. On average, one person a day dies in a car fire. Prevention is best. Keep your car maintained. Many fires occur because of leaking seals where oil or gas come in contact with hot metal.

If you smell burning rubber or plastic or any smoke, immediately pull over to a safe place and check it out. If a fuse continues to go out, that's a sign of a short. Don't ignore it. Get the car inspected. You should carry a fire extinguisher in your vehicle. If the fire is fueled by your gas line, forget about using it and get a safe distance away. At least 150 feet. Warn others in the area and keep them away while calling 911.

Wildifire: If you become trapped park in an area clear of vegetation. Close all windows and ventilation. Cover yourself with wool blanket or jacket. Lie on the floor. Call 911.

If you are locked in your trunk, either through a carjacking or your friends played a really mean joke on you, do you know how to get out? And get new friends? If the trunk has a release lever, use it. Do you know if yours has one? Where it is? All cars since 2002 should have one. Be calm. Trunks are not airtight. Don't hyper-ventilate. The greater danger is heat or cold, depending on your environment. See what tools you have handy. Trunks are, well, trunks. People put a lot of stuff in them. If the spare is in there, it's likely the tire iron is too. That's an excellent tool and weapon. Escape through the back seat. Some are fold down, which makes it easy. Others don't, but it's easier to tear through material than metal. Use the tire iron to punch through. If none of that works, and you've been car-napped, disconnect the brake and tail lights. You might even be able to reach through and break out the lights. The lack of these lights might lead to someone calling the car in and/or the police pulling you over. Use the tire iron to pry open the trunk itself or at least make an opening to signal for help. If the car is speeding down the highway at 70 miles an hour, that is not the moment to jump from the trunk. Every vehicle must eventually stop for re-fueling, usually at a place where there are people.

Keep two bottles of water and power bars within reach of the driver's seat.

Even though you have four-wheel drive, that doesn't mean the vehicle stops any faster. Physics rules: mass times velocity. In Colorado, I was always amazed to see people flying by in their four-wheel drive vehicles, apparently thinking the traction would remain the same if they had to swerve or suddenly brake.

When you start seeing cars that have slid off the road, that's a sign. Black ice is a great danger. You can't see it. The largest warning sign you will get of it is other cars off the road. Slow down.

If you skid, turn into the skid to straighten out.

People have a panic response to not being able to the drive their car. During any moderate to extreme emergency you will quickly see long line of people with gas cans, desperate to get gas. Wouldn't it be so much easier to have that fuel already stored? I keep at least 20 gallons of gas, in 5 gallon containers, at my home. I use StaBil in it and rotate on a set schedule.

Consider what range your emergency supply can take you?

When I take trips longer than a day, I take spare gas with me.

Never, ever, use gas to start a fire. A neighbor on Hilton Head died trying to start a fire on the beach using gas. It's faster than you are.

PLANE CRASH

If you have to evacuate, LEAVE all your stuff. I start with that because every runway emergency I've watched where they evacuate the plane, people are bringing their briefcases, purses, and even carry-ons. LEAVE IT.

First, let's stay in reality. The odds of dying in a car crash are 1 in 98 for a lifetime. In a plane crash: 1 in 7,178. Some of that is because you spend more time in a car than in a plane (unless you work as a pilot). Still, flying is much safer than driving.

Nevertheless, let's cover safety issues with planes.

Where to sit? Statistics from crashes indicate it's safest to sit in the rear of the plane. Yes, I know it takes longer to get on and off, but that's what the numbers show. Despite that, I prefer to be near an exit. I'll take the exit row every time, and not just for the extra room.

What to wear? There is a reason military flight crews wear a specific outfit. It's because the greatest danger is flame. Wear long pants, a long sleeve shirt, and shoes you can move quickly in: ie, don't be doing the Hawaiian shirt, shorts and sandals.

Keep your seat belt fastened at all times. Flight attendants will tell you horror stories of abrupt, unexpected turbulence that bounced them off the ceiling of the plane.

If the oxygen masks drop, put yours on before helping others.

What is the safest airline to fly? Because crashes are so few, statistics don't help you here. For me, the key element is the pilot, not the plane or airline. I prefer military trained pilots.

What is the most important thing to know? Where the closest exit is. Yes, turn and look behind you. Orient yourself to the plane. They put that safety lighting along the aisles in after learning that in the smoke and confusion of a crash, people quickly became disoriented.

What about other passengers? Before 9-11, a pilot friend told me his largest safety concern was not the plane, the weather, etc, it was the passengers. He was right. There is a person who did not get on one of the fatal planes that day because she just didn't feel right about the people she saw boarding.

What is your safety role? Pay attention. Realize pilots can't see the plane behind them. In the case of British Midland Flight 092, this was key. I cover the events leading up to this crash in *Stuff Doesn't Just Happen I: The Gift of Failure*. Briefly, the pilots had smoke in the cockpit. In the rear of the plane, passengers saw smoke and flame coming out of one engine. However, the pilots believed the smoke was coming from the other engine (air conditioning units on an upgraded model had been switched from one engine to another). So they shut down the wrong engine. By the time they realized their mistake, it was too late. When passengers saw the wrong engine shut down, they should have notified the flight crew. Never assume the experts know what they're doing!

Listen to the safety briefing. Yes, I know you've heard it a million times. But it's called a safety briefing for a reason. It will also give you an idea of the level of safety-consciousness of the crew.

When evacuating the plane, get away from it. At least five hundred feet upwind of the plane. Burning fuel is the most dangerous element after a crash.

You laugh every time they show how to buckle and unbuckle your seat belt. Wait until you have to do it in the midst of flame and smoke. Some people will forget. Also, if you are helping someone else, you need to know how to do it.

Remove sharp objects from your body before crashing. Yes, I know the TSA has already done most of that, but that pen in your breast pocket could be your own vampire stake.

If your plane crashes in a remote area, should you stay with the plane or not? Stay. Most planes have a transponder. And it's easier to find a crash site than you wandering in the wilderness. Shift into scavenge mode, using the plane as the source.

TRAIN CRASH

Once more, if you see a problem, contact the crew immediately. Don't assume they know about it.

Train stations are tempting sites for terrorist attacks because they concentrate people in a closed facility (especially if underground). Stay away from the most crowded section. Don't stand near the edge of the platform. Make sure you know where the exits are. Not only the doors, but most trains have roof emergency exits and windows that also work that way.

Understand whether the track is electrified or not. The simple rule is if there is a third rail, it's the one with the juice in it. Don't go near it unless you've just hijacked *Pelham 123* and are about to get caught and don't want to go to the slammer for life.

Ride toward the rear of the train. Most collisions are head on. The further back you are, the better. Remember, though, that a collision will mean you're thrown forward. Since trains don't have safety belts, check what is in front of you. Do you want to hit that?

If you survive the crash, get away from the crash site, but get in contact with emergency services. If in a tunnel, most have emergency walkways. Do not walk on the tracks. Not only because of the possibility of electrocution, but another train might be coming.

While it was cool in *Stand By Me*, don't cross trestles.

Do you have train tracks near your house? Be especially aware if they are on a downhill run with a curve. Prime area for a train to run off the tracks. Hopefully your house isn't in the path, but also be aware that toxic cargo is often carried by rail. If ordered to evacuate because of a train accident/derailment, do so.

BOAT, FERRY, CRUISE SHIP, ETC.

When boating, ALWAYS wear your life jacket, even though it might not be required by law. When would we need a life jacket? In case of an accident. But the very nature of the word 'accident' means it would be an unexpected situation. What good is the life jacket we're not wearing?

The rules of boating safety:

Be weather-wise. Always check local weather. Watch the skies. Better to be safe then dead.

Follow a pre-departure checklist. Make sure you have all the safety gear required.

Designate who is in charge.

Don't speed.

Let someone know where you are going and how long you plan to be gone.

Avoid alcohol.

Learn to swim. Check all passengers to determine who does and doesn't know how to swim.

Taking the ferry back and forth from Whidbey Island made me think about and research this topic. Also, I commanded a Maritime Operations Special Forces Team, so we spent a lot of time in the water. I also graduated the

Royal Danish Navy's Fromankorpset Combat Swim School.

Those experiences taught me that I like hot tubs and otherwise not getting wet.

Don't take a cruise. Joking (not), but they said the *Titanic* was unsinkable. But if you do decide to take a cruise, pay attention to the safety briefings. Even before that, book on a line that has a good safety record. Consider the make-up of the crew. Ever notice how in most cruise ship disasters the crews are the first one off? And most don't speak your language?

Know where the closest flotation devices are. Know how to put them on.

Know where the closest life rafts are. How do they get from ship to water?

Do you know what the evacuation signal is via the ship's horn? Seven short blasts followed by one long, followed by get the heck off the boat.

If you have the time, layer your clothing before putting on your life vest. This will help keep you warm. Most of the Titanic deaths occurred from freezing in the water. If you are in cold water, keep moving. It will keep you warm. Don't just sit there in your vest. Kick your legs, splash your arms.

If you have to jump into very cold water, expect to be shocked. Literally. Cold shock can cause you to involuntarily take a deep breath, and if you're underwater, fill your lungs with water. Keep your mouth shut until you surface. Then yell "FRAK!"

Know where you are on the ship. Take the time to walk the path from your cabin to the deck several times. Consider what it will be like making that trip in the dark and in smoke. Count the number of turns and which direction so you can do it blindfolded. Take the quickest route, not the shortest. Do not take an elevator. Have a route to both sides of the ship in case it starts to list.

TALL BUILDING

Ever heard of base jumping? There were times going out of the back of an MC-130 Combat Talon, where I know we were jumping below 500 feet. Do you work or live in a tall building? Do you have a way to get out if an entire floor below you is impassable?

A parachute might be one way. If you have one. And if you can get through a window. Often, in skyscrapers, these are made of practically unbreakable material.

Most people think of the roof. Remember, during 9-11, no one was rescued from the roofs of either of the towers. There are several reasons for that, but mainly the updraft from the fires made landing impossible. Do you even know what the roof of your building looks like? Are there antennas and cell phone transmitters all over it? Again, we go back to conducting an area study. Have you actually gone down all the stairwells in your building? Checked them out?

POWER OUTAGE

We've all experienced a power outage. The country's electrical infrastructure is in poor shape. Also, it's a tempting target for terrorists. With computers controlling more and more of the electrical grid, a simple virus could cripple large parts of the country.

Are you ready?

Beyond the tips already given for preparation, here are specifics to dealing with a power outage:

Cook perishable foods first. Of course, you can only do that if you have that secondary cooking source, which was covered under equipment.

Do you have a backup method for heating and cooling? For heating, a fireplace works. If you have propane in a tank, can you start your fireplace or heating systems without electricity? Do you know how to work the pilot light? For cooling, there are portable fans that are battery powered, but they have limited life. Have you considered getting a generator? A whole house generator that kicks in automatically when the power goes out. If you use a generator, cut power outage down to the absolutely essential: refrigerator and heating and cooling at the margins. Turn off all unnecessary power users.

While we love our Kindles and our Nooks and iPads, have some print material around to read. Things called books.

Use your crank/solar power radio for the latest news.

You've kept your computer backed up on a consistent basis either to the cloud and/or, preferred, to an external hard drive?

Have a landline. They don't require electricity to operate. But make sure all your landline phones don't require to be plugged in to work. Have a basic phone that you can plug into a jack and it will work.

Put luminescent stickers or pieces of glow tape on your light sources so you can find them in the dark.

Do NOT use gas grills or stoves inside. They release carbon monoxide and can cause death.

Make sure your generator is properly wired and vented if you have one.

Close the curtains to keep heat or cool in. Also, remember, a basement will be the most consistent in terms of temperature.

FIRE

Prevention is the most important thing. Here are keys:

If you use a portable heater, turn it off when you leave the room.

Make sure children understand the danger of lighters, matches and fire. Keep fire starters secure.

Never smoke in bed.

Keep flammable objects at least three feet from heat sources.

When frying, boiling or grilling, always stay in the kitchen.

When simmering, baking, roasting or boiling food, remain in the home and check regularly.

Keep anything that can catch fire (over mitts, wood utensils, etc) away from the stove top.

If you have a grease fire, smother it by putting a lid over the pan and turning off the burner.

For an oven fire, turn off the oven and keep the door closed.

Never use your oven to heat your home.

If you have a fireplace, make sure you keep a screen in front of the fire.

Make sure your chimney is swept and cleaned out once a year.

Never plug in more than one heat producing appliance to an outlet.

Make sure your dryer has a lint filter and keep it clean.

Check your outdoor vent flap to make sure your dryer is venting properly. If it's taking longer than usual for clothes to dry, clean lint out of the vent pipe.

Never heat a baby bottle in the microwave, since they heat things unevenly.

For escape planning: Draw a map of the house showing all doors and windows. Make sure everyone knows the plan and how to get out of every room. Make sure everyone knows to meet up at the IRP once they are out.

Practice your evacuation twice a year, once at night. Everything is different in the dark.

Children need to know how to escape on their own.

If your clothes catch on fire, Stop-Drop-Roll, to put the fire out.

Close doors behind you as you leave.

If you touch a door handle and its hot, or the door itself is hot, don't open that door.

Once out, do not go back in.

If you're trapped inside the house, stay in a room with the doors closed. Place a wet towel under the door opening and call 911. If you have a window, open it and wave something colorful or use a flashlight at night.

If you have to escape through smoke, go low, under the smoke.

If you use a fire extinguisher remember the acronym PASS:
Pull the pin and hold the extinguisher facing away from you.
Aim low. Point the extinguisher at the base of the fire.
Squeeze the handle.
Sweep the extinguisher from side to side until the fire is out.

Smoke alarms should be installed on every level of the house, inside every bedroom, and outside sleeping areas. Let children hear what it sounds like when it goes off and what that means and what they need to do. Check your alarms once a month by pressing the test button. Replace batteries at least once a year. Replace alarms every ten years.

Carbon monoxide monitors are not replacements for smoke alarms. One should be emplaced in a central location on every floor of the house. Never use a generator, grill, stove, anything that gives off smoke, inside your house.

BURGLARY

Here are some sobering numbers.

Odds your home will be burglarized this year	1 in 36
Average loss per break-in	$2,230
65% of break-ins occur between 6 am and 6 pm while people are at work	
34% of burglars enter through the front door	
Only 13.6% of burglaries result in an arrest	

Often burglars case a place by doing work such as painting, carpet cleaning, or furniture deliveries. Did you see how the exterminators in *Breaking Bad* had the perfect set up? People would literally hand them the keys to their house, allow them to go through the entire place, make copies of the keys and then the owners would wonder who burglarized them weeks later. Be very, very careful who you allow into your house. To the point of leaning heavily toward paranoia. You might irritate some people, but the list of those who let the wrong person in and paid the price is long.

As an emergency goes from mild, to moderate, to extreme, you have to focus more on survival and less on being the nice person. And there are times, in day-to-day normal life, where being a nice person can be very costly. That is just a reality, with no judgment passed on it.

A burglar can case the outside of your place and get a good idea of what's inside. Not just the house itself and the neighborhood, but your landscaping, the toys your kids leave scattered about, the type of car parked in the driveway.

Newspapers piled up in the driveway are a lighthouse for thieves. They can also leave a fast food/pizza delivery/cleaning flyer jammed in your front door and see how long it stays there. It takes a couple of days to suspend newspaper delivery, so for any trip you are taking, plan that ahead of time. Or have a friendly neighbor come by each day.

If it snows and you are out of town, while your neighbor might not want to shovel your walk, ask them to at least tramp up to the door and drive in your driveway to leave tracks. It makes it look like someone might be there, even someone too lazy to shovel their walk.

If you have glass in your front door, check to see if the alarm system pad is visible through it. If it is, change it or make sure you block the view when arming and disarming.

Thieves knock. Yes, they will ring the doorbell and if you answer, pretend to be something else: asking directions, to clean your gutters, etc. They might carry a clipboard or wear a uniform. Watch anyone who does this and see if they go to your neighbor's house. Let them know you're watching. They don't like to be watched. Write down license plate numbers.

Don't hide stuff in your sock drawer. Really. Once more, think like the other guy. They hit all the obvious hiding places fast. The first room burglars go to is the master bedroom.

There's a method to the way a professional burglar works and you can find that information elsewhere in case you're looking for a new career. But think counter-intuitively if you want a hide spot. Remember, you might lock everything in that fireproof lockbox, but since they can take it with them, it's not a deterrent. You have to put it somewhere not easily found, but where you can grab it quickly on the way out in an emergency.

In Special Forces we often had to consider deterrence to attacks. Opportunistic attackers like thieves go for the easier target. The harder you make your house as a target, the less likely you are to be robbed. Check out your neighbors. Are you a harder target than them? Sort of like when you and your camping buddies are getting chased by the grizzly. You don't have to out-run the grizzly, you just have to out-run your buddies.

Don't overdo it though. Leaving all your lights on and the TV blaring for the two weeks you're trekking the Amazon is indicating to people that no one is home.

Use deadbolts. Regular locks are very easy to get past.

A dog door can be invitation into your house. A dog isn't. I'm a big fan of dogs. Thieves just don't want to mess with them, even though Cool Gus here, snoring at my feet, isn't exactly dangerous looking. Until he gets riled with all 100 pounds and barking.

The two most effective deterrents: a dog and/or a nosy neighbor.

Thieves rarely go into kids' rooms when in the house.

Big windows invite people to look in. They can case your house from the outside. Close curtains in the evening.

Don't use social media to announce your vacation. Every time I see someone tweet "I'm at Starbucks on Elm Street" I have to resist the urge to tweet: "I'm in your home robbing you."

Have your car keys on your nightstand. If someone breaks in, hit the alarm on the keys and your car will act as a poor man's home alarm. In the same manner, when approaching or leaving your vehicle, especially in indoor garages, have the keys in hand.

ROBBERY

This is when you are confronted outside of your home and someone wants to take something of value from you, whether it be your wallet, purse, watch, car, etc.

The rule is simple: give it up.

You are more valuable than any material object.

The most important thing is to remain calm and don't panic. Remember, the robber is often in a turbulent emotional state and could be under the influence of drugs or alcohol. Your panic could add to their panic.

Make eye contact while you agree to comply. Move slowly. Hand over whatever they want. Do not act overly weak or aggressive. Try to remember as much about them as possible. Let them get away, then call 911.

CAR-JACKING

Most car-jackings occur when the vehicle is parked and within five miles of your home. Again, always have your keys ready when approaching or leaving your vehicle. If threatened to give up the keys, give them up. It isn't worth it.

A common plot for carjackers is to bump your car from the rear. When you get out to investigate, they take your car. Let them have it.

Here are some rules of the road:

Don't park in isolated or places where you can't be seen.

Always have your keys ready.

Remember the alarm button on your key fob. Many people forget it in the panic. Consider it your personal alarm system when in range of the car. Test it and see how far away it works.

Look at other cars near yours as you go to it. Be aware of anyone just sitting there. Walk away if someone is.

Don't help the guy with the cast on his arm trying to load his couch into a van. His name was Ted Bundy.

Don't be hesitant to ask for a security escort to your car at a mall, college, etc. People are paid or volunteer to do that.

Be aware. Tune in to the environment. You should never talk or text while driving, don't be on the phone or text while heading to your car.

As Gavin DeBecker wrote in *The Gift of Fear*, if your senses alert to someone or something, trust your instincts and get away.

As you approach your car, check around it, under it, and always, always look in the back seat or cargo compartment of your SUV/minivan.

Always lock your doors once you're in the car.

When stopping at a light, always leave enough room in front of you that you can turn hard and accelerate away if you have to. Don't trap yourself.

If bumped in traffic by a pair of males, be very suspicious. Pull to a lighted, populated place before unlocking your car.

Again, if confronted by a carjacker, don't resist. Get out of the car and let them have it.

Don't chase the robber.

Never agree to be kidnapped. Hit the alarm, drop the keys and run while yelling loudly.

If you are forced to drive, you can crash the car near a busy intersection to attract attention.

CIVIL UNREST AND RIOTS

This can quickly become an extreme emergency on a local or large-scale level. The psychology of crowds is very interesting, but suffice it to say people act very differently when in groups and especially when scared and/or angry.

To get through the initial stages of a riot, you must learn how to survive your fellow human beings.

Be prepared by:

Know the area where you live, work, and go to school. Know alternate routes.

Get familiar with the area. Check maps by looking at your phone apps.

If you can prepare and have to travel through an area that might have a riot, carry a solution for rinsing your eyes out in case of tear gas.

Make sure you have identification.

When traveling, aim for as many crossroads as possible because they give you three options for directions.

Remain calm.

Hide. Avoidance is always best.

Blend in while moving away. Avoid law enforcement if they have donned their riot gear because they will tend to arrest first and ask questions later.

If you must pass through rioters/looters/etc. wear long sleeves, long pants, consider a motorcycle or other helmet.

Walk, don't run, as you might attract attention. Don't make eye contact. Don't confront people. Don't stop. If you're with someone from your team, hold hands tightly.

Don't get involved. It's not your riot.

Stay close to walls, on the edges of crowds. Avoid bottlenecks.

If you're in your car, don't stop. You are in a position of power as long you keep moving, slowly but surely. Don't speed up or act aggressive. People will give way. Keep your doors locked and your windows up.

Riots usually happen on streets, not in buildings. Get off the street and into a building. Stay away from windows. Look for another exit. Be careful of fire.

If necessary, on foot, go with the flow. Become part of the crowd and edge your path away from the violence.

TERRORIST ATTACK

Since there are so many ways terrorists can attack, it's hard to be comprehensive. The most common, however, is commonly called the suicide bomber. I believe that's a misnomer. If they were true suicide bombers they'd go out into the middle of the desert and blow themselves up. When they detonate around other people, they are homicide bombers. You have to expand this concept: the terrorists on 9-11 were homicide bombers, using the airplanes as bombs.

The best defense against terrorism is making the target difficult to attack. In fact, our intelligence community and military are doing an outstanding job given the lack of attacks on our country. It's not an issue of what you see in the movies where the hero catches the bad guy just before the bomb goes off, but stopping the bad guy from even being able to emplace the bomb in the first place. It's called hardening the target.

The best defense is citizens being aware.

Here are some keys to counter-terrorism for you to keep in mind:

Reconnaissance. Targets have to be cased. All those tourists snapping happy pictures? What about the one that's taking pictures of security cameras and police positions?

Supplies. While you're preparing for survival, a terrorist is preparing for an attack. Timothy McVeigh had to buy a lot of fertilizer to make the bomb he detonated. Also, think of all those sites where you can buy FBI/DEA/Police jackets, badges, etc.

Training. Yes, the 9-11 pilots were trained by Americans.

Information. When someone asks too many questions about things that shouldn't be talked about, like security, that's a warning.

Rehearsal. Just as you conduct your survival rehearsals, terrorists tend to rehearse their actions. Pay attention to people acting suspiciously.

Top targets for homicide bombers: subways, train and busses. Malls. Restaurants and night clubs. Stadiums. Movie theaters. Schools. Churches. Places where people gather together tightly. Whenever you are in such a place, you should always be aware of where the nearest exit is. Actually, any time you're indoors, you should always know where the exits are. That knowledge can save your life. Think if the power goes off, a fire starts, someone begins shooting. In the panic, it's hard to do what you should have done upon first entering the place.

Be aware. Those warnings not to leave your luggage unattended in the airport are serious. If you see someone walk away from a bag, that's something you shouldn't ignore.

If you are ever in a hostage situation, realize that when the good guys break in to free you, they're going to cuff everyone until they can sort out who is who. A trick kidnappers can play is to tape toy guns to hostages' hands, or pretend to be hostages themselves in order to escape. Let the experts do their job.

If you are at home and hear of a terrorist attack nearby, stay at home. Do not go out. Listen to reliable media sources.

A homicide bomber is carrying a bomb. That sounds self-explanatory, but you need to consider where the bomb is. If it's a vest, they will appear unnaturally bulky. If someone is wearing a coat or jacket that is inappropriate to the weather, that's a warning sign. If they're carrying it in a backpack, briefcase, etc. they often will clutch it to their chest just prior to detonation.

If a bomb goes off, be aware that a common ploy is to have follow on bombs designated to kill the first responders. Do not gather in the area unless you are helping those injured, and even then, be aware there could be secondary or follow on attacks.

While it is best to run away, as a last ditch effort, an effective way to disrupt a homicide bomber is to go low and take their legs out from under them. It is an instinct that a person will put out their hands to break their fall, thus releasing the detonation switch. Unless it's a dead man's switch in which case releasing it makes it go off. It's pretty much a sucky situation all around and you can only do the best you can.

The best defense against terrorism is not the TSA or even the intelligence services. It is aware citizens who pay attention to their surroundings.

ACTIVE SHOOTER

The odds you will be caught in an active shooter emergency are very, very low. Like shark attacks, they tend to gather a lot of news, despite being rare.

Nevertheless, it remains a large concern for many people so we'll cover it.

Understand that it takes a while for law enforcement to respond. Also, do you know what real gunfire actually sounds like?

The first thing is to be aware and to accept pretty much anything is a possibility. It should be standard for you to always be aware of at least two exits when you are inside any place. This is true for a number of possible emergencies. Remember, people will tend to rush toward the way they came in, even if there is a closer exit.

If an active shooting situation develops:

Remember these three words: RUN. HIDE. FIGHT.

If you can, evacuate. Leave regardless of what others want to do. Leave everything behind, just like escaping a plane. Help others escape if they want to come, but do not move wounded people. Keep your hands visible as you exit so police can see you are not armed. Follow the instructions of the police, no matter what they tell you to do. If they tell you face down on the ground, get face down on the ground. There is a good chance you will be cuffed.

If you can't evacuate: If you are in a hallway, get into the nearest room.

Secure the door in the room. Lock it and blockade it with the heaviest objects you can place against it. Silence your cell phone. Turn off any other sources of noise. Hide behind large objects (desks, filing cabinets, etc.).

Remain quiet.

Call 911. If you can't talk, leave the phone on so the dispatcher can listen.

If, as a last resort, you must take action, act aggressively and without reserve. Throw whatever is handy, scream and charge. Take them down.

Understand how law enforcement will be reacting.

They will usually assault in teams. They could be wearing a variety of uniforms, since they might be responding from different agencies. They might use gas, flash-bangs, and other non-lethals to secure an area.

Do not have anything in your hands. Keep your hands visible at all times. Don't make any quick movements. If they are passing you by, searching for the shooter, move in the direction they came from. Remember, the initial breaching team will not stop to provide assistance to wounded. They are going for the shooter. Medical personnel will be following. If you are able, help the medical personnel as they arrive.

If you can, provide police or the dispatcher with the following information:

Location of the shooter. Number of shooters. Description of shooter. Number and type of weapons. Number and location of victims.

Once you are out, you will be held in an area until the situation is under control. Do not leave until instructed.

FIREARMS

I leave this until last because it is rather controversial. I believe a gun is a tool. In itself, it is neither good or bad. It is in how it is used that makes that distinction.

Many survivalists think of weapons before anything else. There is a fundamental question you must answer before going any further: are you willing to use a weapon on another human being?

If the answer is absolutely not, then there's no point reading this section any further.

In the Special Forces Qualification Course, during survival training, you had to kill a small animal. There were some who could not bring themselves to do it. If they weren't willing to do that, they really were in the wrong place.

However, I do believe that most of us are not really aware of the lengths we will be willing to go to in order to save ourselves and those we care about.

We spent a lot of time in Special Forces discussing weapons. Two of the twelve men on an A-Team were Weapons Sergeants. If I make any recommendations here, there are many people who would disagree with my choices, so I'm just going to give an overview.

First, it's not just the gun you have to consider. The same gun with two different bullets is essentially a different weapon. A tendency is to think "bigger is better". I prefer to think accurate is better. Remember, you're not throwing the gun at the target: it's the bullet.

For a survival arsenal here is what I suggest:

A pistol for each team member. All same caliber. While many scoff at 9mm, I see no problem with that as you can carry a lot of rounds and also have a number of rounds in your magazine. Have a holster that can secure the weapon. Secure the holster to you. Carry at least two back-up magazines, ready for use. Get hollow point or similar bullets that make the gun more potent.

A semi-automatic rifle designed for military use. The staple is the AR-15, the civilian version of the M-16. You can spend thousands of dollars outfitting it with laser aiming, telescopic sites, etc. etc. Whatever you do, make sure you can fire it accurately. It is illegal to have an automatic weapon and I was never a fan of firing on automatic anyway. It wastes ammunition and unless you are highly trained, is very inaccurate. Again, carry several loaded back up magazines. I am not a fan of the AK-47, but it's the most prolific gun in the world. Another thing about the AR-15 is that since so many people have them, and the military uses versions of it, ammunition will be easier to scavenge.

A .22 survival rifle. You can stockpile thousands of rounds for this and it's good for hunting. Some of these break down in a way that make them easily transportable, such as the Henry Arms AR-7.

You can consider having a shotgun, but how much can you really carry? A shotgun is useful for home defense though as you don't have to be as accurate and it tends to make a bigger impression on whoever you point it at.

Which brings up this issue: if you point a weapon at someone, you must be prepared to use it. Again, my recommendation is discretion is the better part of valor. A weapon should only be used when your life, or the lives of your team members are at stake and you cannot escape.

NUCLEAR WEAPONS AND ACCIDENTS

Three Mile Island. Chernobyl. Have you heard of them?

Do you live near a nuclear plant? I didn't realize there was one nearby in North Carolina until I was flying in to Raleigh-Durham Airport and saw the cooling tower.

Here is a list of nuclear power reactor sites:

List of nuclear power plants:
http://www.nrc.gov/reactors/operating/map-power-reactors.html

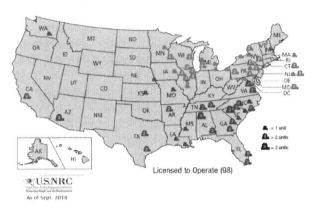

U.S. Operating Commercial Nuclear Power Reactors

Licensed to Operate (98)

U.S.NRC

As of Sept. 2018

What's really scary about that list is to note how old they are.

There are many more nuclear facilities than just reactors. When I lived in Boulder, Colorado, the glow from Rocky Flats south of town was always enchanting. The Savannah River Site in South Carolina? And since I wrote a bestselling series on Area 51, do you know what's just west of there? The Nevada Test Site is where we tested most of our nukes.

So what to do, other than move far, far away?

Let's focus on a meltdown as I'll cover a nuclear explosion later.

Nuclear power plants work by using heat from the reaction to convert water into steam, which powers generators. They produce around 20% of our country's electricity. Over three million Americans live with ten miles of a nuclear plant. That radius is important because emergency response plans have two zones. One is the ten-mile radius where people can be hit by direct radiation exposure. The other is a fifty-mile radius where radiation can contaminate water supplies, crops and livestock.

Without getting into physicist speak, here are the basics: radiation is the danger. Even if you are a distance from the plant, radiation can get into the air through venting or explosion. You want to avoid exposure from material on the ground, from inhaling it, or ingesting it.

Here are the keys to minimize your exposure:

Distance. Get away. The further you are from the source of the radiation, the better. If it is going into the air, check prevailing wind patterns. If you want some history on this, check out how Chernobyl dispersed radiation across Russia and Europe.

Shielding. Put heavy, dense, material between you and the source of the radiation. That is why paper works well. Hunker down in the middle of a library. Or a records center.

There are a series of alerts, curiously named mostly to prevent panic, that you should be aware of it you live near a reactor:

Notification of Unusual Event: a minor problem has occurred but no radiation has leaked or is expected to leak. We're just notifying you because the law says so and we don't want to scare you. But no action on your part is necessary.

Alert: A small problem has occurred and small amounts of radiation have or may leak inside the facility. This won't affect you—we hope—and you don't have to do anything. Personally, I'd be bugging out. Because they are, in essence, telling you thcy've had a breach of containment. They wouldn't be telling you that unless absolutely necessary.

Site Area Emergency: Thcy're a little vague on this one. Area sirens may sound. Listen to your radio or television for safety info. I'd be listening to the radio while leaving.

General Emergency: Radiation could be coming off the plant site. Sirens are sounding. Dogs are barking. Frogs are falling from the sky. Tune to radio/TV for information. I'd check the information first, before bugging. Because you might be better off hunkering down inside your house than going through a radiation cloud.

Measures to be taken in a nuclear emergency:

If trapped keep windows closed in your house and car. Use re-circulating air.

If you are advised to stay in your house, turn of the air conditioner, ventilation fans, furnace and any other air intakes into the house. Go to the basement or other underground area.

If you have been exposed to nuclear radiation take off all clothing. Bag it and seal it. Don't ever wear it again. Safely dispose of as soon as possible. Take a thorough shower. You are literally washing radiation off you. Put fresh, unexposed clothing on. Any exposed food should be disposed of.

Nuclear Weapons

Duck and cover. How many remember that?

A nuclear attack could be limited to a single explosion or a World War.

Let's focus on what you should do:

First, a nuclear war probably won't happen in a vacuum. Keep an eye on the news. It is more likely there could be a small yield nuclear explosion by terrorists and that will probably be a 'dirty' bomb where the fallout will be more dangerous than the initial explosion.

We have DEFCON levels, which are defense readiness conditions for the Armed Forces.

DEFCON 5: lowest state of readiness. Supposed to be the norm.

DEFCON 4: Increased intelligence watch and strengthened security measures. Above normal readiness, but no running around screaming in the streets yet.

DEFCON 3: Increase in force readiness. This is when alerts go to military forces to up their alert status. The Air Force is on 15 minutes notice to mobilize. Still no running around screaming but take some deep breaths.

DEFCON 2: The next step will be nuclear war. All military units are ready to engage in six hours. Start screaming.

DEFCON 1: Nuclear war is imminent. The code name for this is Cocked Pistol, which gives you an idea.

We've never gone to DEFCON 1. Publicly, we've gone to DEFCON 2 once, during the Cuban Missile Crisis. On 9-11, we went to DEFCON 3.

Analyze the intelligence available to you, make a decision whether it's best to stay put or evacuate. Again, this goes to the issue: do you live near a likely target? Military posts? Missile silos? Transportation hub? City? Centers of government? Should you get away? Do you have a place to go? You might have to go further than your hide site.

In *Panic in the Year Zero*, Ray Milland and his family see the mushroom cloud over Los Angeles in the rear view mirror, which is their first clue of the attack. It's better than seeing it through your front windshield. At least they were heading in the right direction.

There are different types of nuclear weapons.

Fission (atomic bombs) are pretty basic and what we are most familiar with. Fusion (hydrogen bombs) are much more powerful. These are also known as thermonuclear weapons because a high temperature is needed to fuse the deuterium and tritium.

For a single nuclear event, which is a distinct possibility (I'm actually rather amazed that a nuclear weapon has not been used since the end of World War II), you will probably get little to no warning.

Again, assess the likelihood of it occurring near you. My estimate is that the most likely terrorist target will be a port, as the weapon will be in a cargo container.

One sign that a nuke has gone off somewhere is the EMP effect. If all electronic devices suddenly fail, assume a nuclear bomb has been detonated high in the atmosphere and expect more to be coming.

If a nuke goes off, seek shelter immediately. The first sign of an explosion will be a flash, which travels at the speed of light. Behind the flash comes the shock wave, so you will have some moments to react. Do not look in the direction of the blast. If outdoors, seek a depressed area, exposing as little of your skin as possible. If indoors, get away from windows and fight the temptation to look to see what the bright light was about—the imploding window will likely kill you with lacerations.

Most people who survive will want to flee. However, this is the exact wrong thing to do. You are exposing yourself to fallout by fleeing. The blast has thrown a large amount of irradiated debris into the air. This fallout will be coming down. You don't want it to come down on you. Your goal is to place the most protection between you and the fallout and radiation. Ideally be underground.

Fallout tapers off relatively quickly. After an hour it's down about 50%. After a day it can be down to only 20%. So these first hours are critical.

After that, the issue is whether this has been a large-scale attack or a local event. If a local event, wait for responders.

INFECTIOUS DISEASES AND BIOLOGICAL/CHEMICAL WEAPONS AND ACCIDENTS

The Black Death killed between 75 to 200 million people between the years 1346-1353. In just seven years. There have been pandemics throughout history and we are due for another one.

A pandemic is an epidemic of infectious disease that spreads across a large region; usually multiple continents. Experts believe the odds of a pandemic within the next fifty years are very high.

Estimates are that:

1 billion people would get sick.

165 million will die

There will be a global recession and depression Why are the odds of a pandemic high? Global population has increased dramatically. People are moving to crowded, central locations: cities. World-wide travel is much faster and more common.

A pandemic will most likely consist of a virus. Viruses are tiny organisms, 100 times smaller than a single bacteria cell. They are an infective agent that typically consists of a nucleic acid molecule in a protein coat that is able to multiply only within the living cells of a host. It needs a host. When a virus infects a host, it invades the cells and take them over in order to carry out its own life process of multiplication and growth.

Anthrax is the most likely agent to be used. It is pretty much 100% deadly when it enters a person's lungs. A minimum fatal dose is one spore and the problem is the symptoms don't show up for days. However, the spores are highly static and tend to clump together and with dust and dirt, making them too big to actually get into the lungs. Thus a package containing anthrax would be very dangerous to the person opening it, or an anthrax bomb deadly for those directly exposed to it, but beyond that immediate circle, others could quickly clear the area and be safe, because it has a very low rate of secondary uptake. This means once it's on the ground, it tends to stay there. So if you are in an area where anthrax is released, go to a sealed room and wait it out. Of more concern is smallpox, because it spreads more easily and is more persistent, although its lethality rate is lower. The problem is that you must quarantine people who are exposed because symptoms might not appear for several weeks.

What are the Six Stages of a pandemic?

The World Health Organization has a Six Stage influenza program, plus two Periods:

Stage 1 No animal influenza virus circulating among animals have been reported to cause infection in humans.

Stage 2 An animal influenza virus circulating in domesticated or wild animals is known to have caused infection in humans and is therefore considered a specific potential pandemic threat.

Stage 3 An animal or human-animal influenza reassortant virus has caused sporadic cases or small clusters of disease in people, but has not resulted in human-to-human transmission sufficient to sustain community-level outbreaks.

Stage 4 Human-to-human transmission of an animal or human-animal influenza reassortant virus able to sustain community-level outbreaks has been verified.

According to the WHO, if an influenza pandemic were to emerge today, we could expect:

As people today are highly internationally mobile, the pandemic virus would spread rapidly around the world.

Vaccines, antiviral agents, and antibiotics to treat secondary infections would quickly be in short supply.

Several months would be needed before any vaccine

became available. This is because some pandemic viruses are new ones.

Medical facilities would be overwhelmed.

There would be sudden and potentially considerable shortages of personnel to provide vital community services as the illness became widespread.

Stage 5 The same identified virus has caused sustained community level outbreaks in two or more countries in one WHO region.

Phase 6 In addition to the criteria defined in Phase 5, the same virus has caused sustained community level outbreaks in at least one other country in another WHO region.

LOST PEAK PERIOD Levels of pandemic influenza in most countries with adequate surveillance have dropped below peak levels.

POST PANDEMIC PERIOD Levels of influenza activity have returned to the levels seen for seasonal influenza in most countries with adequate surveillance.

As long as there has been warfare there have been biological weapons. In early days, corpses were used to spread diseases or infect water supplies. Targets of bioweapons aren't just people, but also crops and animals. With advances in genome sequencing, the threat of bioweapons is growing exponentially.

The problem with bioweapons in warfare has always been that they are indiscriminate in their targets. They affect everyone the same. However, the threat of targeted, sequenced, bioweapons means they could attack certain groups of people with specific genetic markers. Also, terrorists often don't care if they die with their victims.

What To Do?

Depending on where you live and how much you travel will determine what your chances of getting infected. If you live in an urban setting, the chances are higher.

Whether it's a pandemic or just the flu, here are basic steps to take:

Cover your nose and mouth with a tissue when you cough or sneeze. Throw it away after use.

Use a mask if you become aware that people are getting sick. Actually, it might look odd seeing those people in airports wearing a mask, but it's a good idea. Better to look a bit foolish than catch something that will make you sick and might possibly kill you.

Wash your hands with soap and water. Use disinfection. One curious fact brought up in *Contagion* was the number of times we touch our faces with our hands.

Stay away from the sick people. That sounds easy, but what if you're a first responder or a health care provider?

Stay away from crowds.

If it's a true pandemic, it's not likely that a hospital is a place to go as it will quickly become overwhelmed with the sick and dying.

The bottom line is to stay aware and isolate yourself and your team as quickly as possible.

Biological and chemical weapons are normally not weapons of choice for the military because they target indiscriminately. Even for terrorists they have a high failure rate because even though they can be very lethal there is the problem of delivery and dispersal. So many variables can affect chemical and biological agents: air quality, winds, temperature, humidity, and the shelf life of the element itself. When you look at biological/chemical agents, you also have to consider accidental release.

Looking at your area study, do you have a level four containment facility for biological agents around the corner from you? Not likely, but what industries are in your area, upwind, or upriver? Are you along a rail, water or road line on which dangerous agents are transported?

One method of dispersal would be of agents via a crop dusting plane. The plane would have to fly quite low, but if you ever see one in a place where there are no crops to dust, seek shelter. A good target for such an attack would be an outdoor sports stadium. Even better, an air show where people expect to see planes and even smoke coming out of a plane.

Another mode of attack would be to put a biological agent into a water supply. This is one reason to have a top-level filtering system in your house and use it for drinking water. Our first priority in our household is to put in a Kinetico system wherever we live. Not only is the water safer, it tastes better.

You can purchase a gas mask, but the problem is you must know when to put it on and how to use it. Many agents also work via your skin, rendering a gas mask ineffective.

Avoidance is the best defense for these kinds of attacks. As noted, targets are places where a large group of people are contained in a tight space. I don't go to movie theaters (watch it on-demand). I don't go to sporting events (can you say *Black Sunday*?). Ditto on air shows. When going shopping, go at off peak times, during the week, rather than on the weekend when malls and stores are most crowded.

If you are at home when there is a chemical/biological attack or accident, shut all air intake into the house: windows, doors, garage. Turn off your heating/air conditioning. You do not want air circulating inside the house or coming in from outside. Choose the room that has the least windows and doors. Run tape along any windows where there are seams. Cover the windows with thick polyethylene sheeting.

You should have one room in the house designated as the safe room to survive the initial stages of a nuclear, chemical or biological incident. When you have all team members and supplies in the room, finish sealing it by taping around the door, paying particular attention to the gap between the bottom of the door and the floor. You can use a wet towel and then tape it over. Look for any air vents (either in or out) and seal those with sheeting.

Specific Natural Threats

TORNADO

Tornados strike with little warning. If an alarm or alert has been sounded, even if you don't see one, assume it's there. Seek shelter. NOW!

Underground is always best for a shelter. Those areas that are prone to tornadoes have designated shelters. If your house is in a tornado area, you should have a room, a neighbor's house with a room, or a shelter already decided upon.

If a shelter is not available, go to the basement of a building. Stay away from windows and glass. Cover yourself with a mattress, cushions, blankets or a sleeping bag. Look around you for objects that could be blown over and don't be in their path if they fall.

If stuck in a building with no basement, go the lowest floor and the smallest room near the center of the house. Or under a stairwell or in an interior hallway with no windows. Bathrooms are good because you have pipes in the wall which help strengthen them and you can lie in the bathtub. Lie on the ground, face down, and cover your head with your hands and arms. If you have a strong table, take cover under that. Cover yourself with cushions, blankets or a mattress.

Stay in your safe place until well after the danger has passed. Have your GnG bag with you with your survival radio so you can check in to the National Weather Service.

When you do leave your shelter, be careful. Avoid power lines and water that might be touched by power lines. Stay clear of buildings as they still might collapse. Avoid using open flame as it's likely there are gas leaks.

HURRICANE

Evacuate.

That sounds so simple, yet just today I read an article while researching about a family killed because they refused a mandatory evacuation for Hurricane Sandy. Their house had been robbed when they evacuated previously and they didn't want that to happen again. What happened this time makes a robbery look like such a not bad thing. Hurricanes, unlike tornados, move slowly. So you will have warning and time to get away.

Most of the preparation for a hurricane you've already done in preparing your house. There are some special actions you can add:

Board and tape windows. Plywood is best for covering window. For taping, use alligator tape, not duct tape. Masking tape is not useful.

Fasten your roof down to the house with tie down straps. Really long ones. You need to have these on hand *before* the hurricane is coming.

Turn off gas and/or propane.

Clear away debris that can be picked up and smash into the house and windows.

Secure all outdoor furniture. If you have a pool, put the furniture into the water.

Make sure your garage doors are closed.

Looking at the deaths from Hurricane Sandy, over half of them were from falling trees/limbs. Make sure the trees around your house are properly trimmed and if old and unstable, pay to have them removed. It's worth your life and your family's lives.

As the storm approaches, turn your freezer and refrigerator to their coldest settings.

Pack any coolers with as much ice as possible. Use them first instead of opening the refrigerator door. If you grew up like I did, your dad was always yelling at your for opening the fridge door anyway.

Fill bathtubs with water.

Make sure all vehicles are topped off.

Know where the closest shelter is for you and for your pets.

If you have to evacuate leave a note saying where you are going.

Unplug everything before leaving.

Turn off electricity, gas and water.

After the hurricane passes, beware of flooding.

Use flashlights or chem lights, never candles.

Do not use tap water after the storm until you are sure it isn't contaminated.

EVACUATE.

If you did not evacuate and it strikes, then you are in tornado mode. Go back a couple of pages ago and do what's listed.

HEAT WAVE AND DROUGHT

Heat waves are becoming more common. In the desert section I listed ways to deal with that environment; dealing with a heat wave in your home and work area can be a regular occurrence depending on where you live.

Keys:

Naturally, keep your air-conditioning at a livable level. However, if there is a power outage or you don't have air-conditioning there are things to keep in mind. Lower floors are always cooler as heat rises. Close shades and lower blinds. Go somewhere that does have air conditioning such as a mall or theater.

Drink sufficient water but don't overdo it. We've covered the danger *over-hydration*.

Eat lighter meals during a heat wave so the body doesn't have work as hard digesting, producing more internal heat. Keep your skin covered. If outdoors, wear a hat to protect from sunlight. Wear lighter colors to reflect sunlight.

Use fans in your house to promote circulation of air. In the evening at night, open windows to let in cooler air, then close them in the morning along with blinds and shades.

Turn off extra sources of heat such as lights and appliances. Don't use the stove or oven.

Avoid alcohol and caffeine as they are diuretics and dehydrate you.

Remember your pets. They also suffer in a heat wave. Put them in the shower. Give them a cool, wet towel to lie on. Make sure they have plenty of water to drink.

Heat waves contribute to drought. It is considered an 'insidious hazard of nature' because it creeps up on you. How it occurs varies by region. Six days without rain is nothing in the desert. In the tropics, that is a drought. The bottom line is a lack of normal precipitation over an extended period of time leads to drought.

Here are ways to deal with drought:

Purchase rain barrels and other ways of collecting rain water. The typical roof produces 500 gallons of run off from just one inch of rain! Typically the water is considered non-potable, but it can be used for a variety of uses, and can be filtered in an emergency.

Make sure the dishwasher and clothes washer are full before using.

Don't leave water running on a faucet. Take shorter showers.

Dishwasher	8 to 12 gallons per load
Clothes washer	50 gallons per load
Shower	3 to 5 gallons per load
Running faucet	2 to 3 gallons per minute

Remember that drought can lead to . . .

WILDFIRE

All fires start small. All fires go out. What matters is what happens in between.

Recently we had a wildfire here in Tennessee that destroyed numerous homes and businesses and killed several people. This followed a couple of months of drought, which should have raised awareness levels higher.

The wind throws embers one mile or more ahead of the flames. These embers start new fires. A fast wild fire has an intense wall of heat in front of it. Even if the flames haven't arrived, it will combust the most flammable material.

As the main fire approaches your house, strong winds blow embers everywhere possible – under decks, against wood fences, into woodpiles, and through open doors and windows.

In some places the air is so smoky that you can't see more than 10 feet.

Close to where the fire is burning most intensely, the air is far too hot to breathe.

The rising smoke and ash create winds on the ground which cause the fires to burn even more intensely.

Fires like this occur every year. Wild fires don't just happen in the summer; in many areas fires can happen year round. When it is dry and windy be watchful and prepare to take action to protect your family and property.

To prepare your home if you live in an area prone to wildfires, here is a list of things to do:

Keep your roof and gutters free of leaves.

Store firewood at least 30 feet away from structures. The nice pile up against the side of your house is called fuel for a wildfire.

Your outdoor furniture should be made of noncombustible materials.

Clear the area around your house of combustible material such as leaves, bark, pine needles and underbrush. Especially trim grass and brush around your propane tank. Optimally you want a hundred foot barrier of no trees, shrubs or bushes around your house.

When building walls, barriers, gates, landscaping, etc use noncombustible materials.

When evacuating a wildfire, you should leave as soon as you receive notice. Considering there is a chance your house might not be there for you to come back to, besides your GnG bag, also take that fireproof container with all your key documents in it. And your pets. Beyond that, forget about it. Just like below, when discussing a tsunami, people are more important than any keepsake. And wild fires move fast!

While evacuating, make sure you have enough gas. This goes back to always keeping your tank at least half full.

Leave any gates open for firefighters and others.

Drive with headlights on. If it's smoky, close all windows, and recirculate air inside the vehicle.

If you get trapped, park in an area that is clear of vegetation (parking lot, gravel area, dirt), close all windows and vents, cover yourself with a blanket or coat and lie on the floor. Car tires may burst from heat.

In an extreme situation, you have to consider whether you can stay in your house only if: your only escape route is blocked; smoke is so thick you can't travel; you don't have time to evacuate; or emergency personnel tell you to.

You cannot stay in your house if: you have wood siding or shingles; you're located in a narrow canyon or on a steep slope; you have a lot of vegetation close around the house. Find a neighbor with a better house.

If you do stay in a house, do the following: use a sprinkler or the sprinkler system to wet the yard. Wet the roof with a hose. Turn off all propane and gas. Close all windows and doors. Move fabric covered furniture away from large windows or sliding doors. Turn off everything that circulates air through the house. Close all interior doors.

On the opposite extreme from wild fires, there is . . .

BLIZZARD

Like a hurricane, there is usually warning before a blizzard strikes. A blizzard is defined as a severe snowstorm with sustained winds over 35 miles per hour and lasting more than three hours.

You're already done the preparation in your home and car. For work/school, with adequate notice, you should be sent home.

Specific preparation when warned of a blizzard:

Stock up on de-icing and salt and sand.

If you have a snow blower, make sure it's working now and topped off.

Check and clean your gutters.
Get your snow shovel out.

EARTHQUAKE

The USGS publishes maps about the potential for earthquakes in the United States and keeps it updated. While every year people in Florida worriedly follow the weather channel and track hurricanes, people in California, Oregon and Washington rarely check on the earthquake likelihood.

There is a 62% chance San Francisco will have a 6.7 or worse earthquake by the year 2032. The Pacific Northwest is long overdue for a major quake.

Preparation and securing your home

No building is earthquake proof. Just like no ship is unsinkable, aka the *Titanic*.

A seismic retrofit usually means securing the house to its foundation if it isn't already. If you take one of the carriage tours in Charleston, SC you'll see bolts sticking out the sides and fronts of old buildings. They've been retrofitted since the earthquake of 1886. Do you know how your building will fare in an earthquake? Where you live? Where you work? For example, in downtown Seattle there are beautiful old brick buildings which, while quite elegant, are a very bad place to be in case of an earthquake.

Besides the building itself, the ground it's on is key. One of my greatest concerns on Whidbey Island looking at the high bluffs that lined the shore. They were sand and dirt, not rock. People who'd lived there for decades told me of constantly eroding bluffs and houses having to be taken off their foundations and moved back inland. Imagine what an earthquake would do to those high bluffs?

Beware of things moving inside the house. Look around. What large items of furniture do you have that aren't secured? That could be tipped over during an earthquake? Look at what you hang on the walls. What happens if that fell off? Think of shelves and what could fall off them. There are entire companies that specialize in earthquake proofing your dwelling, but some common sense can go a long way.

Secure tabletop objects. TVs, stereos, computer monitors, etc. should all be secured.

Make sure your gas appliances have flexible connectors to reduce risk of leak and fire.

Anchor your furniture. When anchoring to a wall, make sure you attach to a stud, not drywall. Purchase a stud finder for this.

Make sure your windows are safety glass or cover them with shatter-resistant film. Make sure you use safety film and not just a sun film.

Ceiling fans and lights should be double secured with a second chain, loose enough to allow them to sway and to keep them from coming completely loose if the primary attachment fails.

Framed pictures and painting should be anchored to a stud and with a closed hook so they can't shake off.

Strap your water heater to a upright wall nearby.

Like every emergency situation covered so far, the best thing you can do is be properly prepared and then be knowledgeable. Consider some special adaptations if you live in a high earthquake zone. Think about how much time you spend in bed? Doesn't it make the odds of an earthquake happening while you are there high? It's a good idea to keep shoes, flashlight and even a bike or construction helmet underneath your bed.

If you're indoors, stay there.

Get under and hold onto a desk or table. Or stand against an interior wall.

Stay clear of exterior walls, glass, heavy furniture, fireplace and appliances.

Stay out of the kitchen.

If in an office building, stay away from exterior walls and glass.

Do not use elevators.

If you're outside, get into the open, clear of buildings, power lines, trees or anything else that can fall on you.

If you're driving, move the car out of traffic and stop. DO NOT park under bridges or overpasses. Get clear of trees, light posts and power lines. If you resume driving, watch out for road hazards, broken levels of roads, and downed power lines.

If you are in a mountainous area, be aware of the potential for landslides.

After an earthquake, watch out for fire hazards. Shut off valves for gas. If electrical wiring is damaged, turn off the main breaker.

If you are near the ocean be aware of . . .

TSUNAMI

If you live in a tsunami zone, any earthquake should be cause for concern. Even one across the ocean.

If the water recedes suddenly, get out. Don't go pick up the flopping fish or you'll end up being one.

If animals start acting strangely, or running away, follow. Animals are often a good indicator that something in nature is abnormal. Often they are smarter than us. They don't grab a flashlight in a horror movie to go investigate that strange noise in the basement.

Evacuate when warned. Right away. Don't stop to gather personal items. Get your GnG and go.

Make sure you have a vehicle route and a walking route to higher ground. In the panic of evacuation, the vehicle route can turn into an obstacle.

Bottom line, get to higher ground. If you can't, climb a large tree, go up the stairs to the roof.

If you are caught in the water, grab onto something that floats. The real danger is being smashed against other objects.

Do not return until officially notified. Sometimes tsunamis come in groups.

VOLCANO

What did your Area Study say? Take a drive through Oregon and you can see all the volcanoes dotting the horizon. A trip up to Crater Lake is really worth it.

There are different types of volcanic eruptions. You have the trickle of lava slowly moving downhill to the violent explosion of an all-out eruption. The good news is most volcanoes are carefully monitored and you should get some warning. In 1980, USGS geologists convinced authorities to close off Mount St. Helens to the public and in doing so saved thousands of lives. Despite that, fifty-seven people were killed. For two months prior to eruption, the mountain gave off serious indications of trouble. If you live near a volcano, what you should do, beyond the regular survival preparations you've already put into place:

Pay attention to the news regarding the state of the volcano. If warnings are being issued, for what kind of eruption are they being issued?

Know your escape routes. Like those in a tsunami zone, plan your vehicle and foot routes. The USGS can provide you with a hazard map around the volcano to help you plan. You should have multiple routes planned because you don't know exactly how the volcano will erupt and in what direction.

Leave immediately if ordered to evacuate. Keep tuned in on your radio for the latest updates.

Get to high ground. Lava follows the rule of gravity.

Don't try to outrun an eruption as the gas flow from an eruption can expand at over 300 miles an hour.

Avoid breathing poisonous gasses. Do not go to low ground as gasses accumulate there.

Beware of roof collapse if a lot of ash is being deposited.

Never try to cross a lava flow even if it appears the surface has cooled and solidified.

Most people die in mudflows and flooding after an eruption. Thus, even though you are out of the immediate danger, be aware of these other dangers.

MUD/LAND SLIDE

When you did your area study, did you focus on the potential for mud or landslides? If you have any steep terrain in your locale, these are always a possibility. Check the history of your area with a Google search and these keywords. In fact, do a Google search of your area connecting it with all potential natural and man-made disasters.

The difference between a mudslide and a landslide is that the former has a higher degree of content. Mudslides can have the consistency of wet concrete and the same effect.

The best preparation is to not build or travel through areas where there is a high likelihood.

Warning signs: Periods of heavy rainfall or snow melt saturate the ground and cause instability in sloped areas. Areas prone to earthquakes, hurricanes, wildfires and other natural disasters are also prone to slides. Roads cut through hills and mountains are susceptible since the natural geography has been disturbed. Locations at the base of steep ridgelines, hills and mountains are in danger.

If you're in a building and notice cracks developing in the walls, that's a sign that trouble is coming. More signs:

If doors and windows begin to get jammed.

Utility lines start to break.

Fences, poles, and trees start to tilt.

Water starts accumulating in abnormal places.

The terrain starts to bulge or starts slanting at the base of the slope.

GET OUT.

DAMS

In your area study, did you find out you live downstream from a dam? There are over 80,000 dams in the United States. About one-third of those pose a danger to life and property if they fail.

While a dam failure can happen catastrophically, without warning, often there are signs that you can heed. Flooding can cause overtopping or a build up behind the dam that exceeds its capacities. One of the events covered in *Stuff Doesn't Just Happen II: The Gift of Failure* is the St. Francis Dam failure which was one of the worst engineering disasters of the 20th Century, just north of Los Angeles. By the way, a dam with the exact same design still exists in LA!

Dams can fail for the following reasons:

Sabotage/terrorism, although a dam is much harder to destroy than you would think.

Structural failure.

Movement in the foundation of the dam; earthquakes are a great danger to dams.

Settlement and cracking of concrete or embankment dams.

Poor maintenance and upkeep.

Make sure you know your evacuation route. Have one for vehicle and one for on foot. Make sure you can do the route in the dark. Disasters rarely conveniently time themselves for us.

Get out of channels below the dams. Most people killed in a dam failure are caught by the massive amount of water being channeled downstream and the debris carried with it.

FLOOD

Floods often happen in conjunction with other events, such as a hurricane or a tsunami. Storm surge can also cause floods, as can extreme rainfall. Our house flooded at 5,600 feet on a ridgeline in Boulder, CO, because the rain overwhelmed the ability of the land to absorb it and the entire water table rose.

Do not under-estimate the power of water. As already noted a gallon of water weighs 8.34 pounds. Think how big a gallon jug is? Consider hundreds of thousands of those jugs, each weighing over 8 pounds, moving. That's power.

Know if you live in a flood plain. Understand what it means when they say 'hundred year flood zone'. Basically, that means in any year, you have at least a 1% chance of the water reaching that level or beyond.

Regardless of your beliefs, the reality is that water levels of the oceans are rising. Storms are becoming more extreme. That is not dogma, but fact. So be prepared.

There are three main types of floods:
Coastal (surge) Flood

Occurs on coast-lines of large bodies of water as the name implies. It is the result of extreme tides caused by severe weather. Storm surge pushes water onto shore. A storm surge timed with a high tide can be devastating.

There are 3 levels:

Minor: some beach erosion but no major damage.

Moderate: more beach erosion and some damage to homes and businesses.

Major: Serious threat to life and property. Large scale beach erosion. Roads will be flooded and structures damaged.

River (fluvial) Flood

This happens when excessive rainfall over a period of time overwhelms a river's capacity to carry the water. It can also be caused by snow melt, ice jams, and debris jams. A dam failure can cause an abrupt and catastrophic form of river flood. And vice versa: a river flood can cause dam and levee failures.

There are two types of river floods:

Overbank flooding is when the water continues to rise.

Flash flooding occurs when there is an intense, high velocity rainfall.

It might not be raining where you are, but the river can flood from rain and run off upstream.

Surface (pluvial) Flood)

This happens separate from an existing body of water. Torrential rainfall overwhelms the area's normal way of channeling water.

There are two types:

Intense rain saturates an urban drainage system and water back flows into streets and structures.

Run off isn't absorbed by the ground and the water level rises.

A flood WATCH means a flood is possible.
A flood WARNING means the flood is happening.

If you have time, move valuables in your house to the highest level before evacuating.

When evacuating, move to higher ground, away from water sources, such as rivers and lakes.

Never go around a barrier on a road during a flood. It's there for a reason. To keep you from being dumb.

If evacuating in your car avoid standing water. Drive very, very slowly. Many people have lost their lives driving into a dip in the road and submerging their vehicle. If you live in a flood zone, prepare your car as I described for the boat/ferry.

Don't walk through moving water. Even very shallow water can knock you off your feet and sweep you into deeper water.

Flash floods kill a lot of people every year. Here are the keys:

Never drive through a flooded road or water flowing over a bridge.

Stay to high ground.

Keep track of weather information. Just because it's not raining where you are, doesn't mean it's not raining up-water.

Do not stay in a flooded car.

If the car is swept away or submerged, stay calm and wait for the vehicle to fill with water. The doors will not open before then (although you might try to get out the sunroof). Open the door, hold your breath, and swim for the surface. You will now be in the current. Point your feet downstream. Go over obstacles, never under. Strive to angle toward dry ground, but don't fight directly against the current.

Here is a valuable video of what do if your car begins to submerge.
It's only 2 minutes long but could save your life:
https://www.youtube.com/watch?v=maywde6eILE&t=8s

If you are stuck above the flash flood, such as in a tree, stay in place and wait for rescue rather than risking the fast-moving water.

SOLAR FLARE/EMP

It's estimated there is a 12% chance Earth will experience a massive mega-flare erupting from the sun in the next decade. This event would be devastating in impact and after-effect.

The last one to strike Earth was the Carrington Event in 1859. When it occurred, northern lights were reported in Honolulu, while southern lights were seen in Santiago, Chile. The flares were so powerful, people could read newspapers at night just from the light of the resulting aurora.

Of more significance, the geomagnetic disturbances were so strong that telegraph operators reported sparks jumping from their keys; some sets even caught on fire. The telegraph networks reported major outages. The Earth's magnetic field was so disturbed, the readings were off the scale.

Without getting into the science, a similar sized eruption now would severely damage the world's power grid, broke pipelines, disrupt GPS satellites and damage, if not wipe out, radio communication.

It's estimated the damage would cost 1 to 2 trillion dollars. Of more concern to you and I is that it would take 4 to 10 years to recover. While that is a worst case scenario, it would essentially mean a breakdown of civilization. That's because with a long term outage, transportation, banking, and government services would crumble. Drinking water would cease to be delivered. Perishable foods and medications would be done.

In 1989, a solar flare collapsed Canada's Hydro-Quebec power grid in 90 seconds and it took nine hours to restore. On 23 July 2012, a massive solar flare twice the power of the one that hit Canada occurred, but missed the Earth.

Electromagnetic Pulse is essentially a high-intensity burst of electromagnetic particles. In the case of the nuke, an EMP nuclear event is actually a more likelier terrorist scenario in my opinion than a physically destructive nuclear blast. What I mean is that for an EMP attack to be effective, the weapon does not need to be detonated inside our borders. A ballistic missile carrying an EMP or a nuclear warhead launched off our coast or from a plane outside our borders could have a devastating effect, especially if it targets large centers, such as New York City.

The EMP blast would seriously disrupt our electronic infrastructure. Power is gone. Which leads to water and sewer systems being gone. Most planes and cars would no longer work (sucks if you're in the air when this happens, and yes I do think about it, along with that gremlin on the wing unscrewing the bolts). Computers would no longer work. All electronic records, unless they are shielded, will be wiped out. Pretty much every usual means of communication would be gone.

There are ways of protecting some equipment from EMP, but if the overall grid has failed, I'm not sure that's of much use. The more important thing is to be prepared for an extreme emergency of long duration where electronics do not function.

The key is that YOU ARE NOW PREPARED!

Beware Scam Artists after a Disaster

Yes, there are those unscrupulous people who will try to take advantage of those whose lives have already been devastated. These are similar to the people you will have to face down after an extreme emergency.

After a disaster, there will be many business, faith-based, community-based, volunteers, government agencies and others who will come forth to try to help. There is a disaster fraud hotline at 866-720-5721.

Here are ways to spot these scam artists and avoid them:

Government workers never charge for their services. They have photo ID.

Do not trust anyone who tells you that you will receive a government payment but asks that you give them an up-front payment first.

There is never a fee to apply for FEMA disaster assistance or receive it. The same for FEMA or US Small Business Administration property damage inspections.

To register for FEMA help call 800-621-3362 or visit www.DisasterAssistance.gov or m.fema.gov from a smartphone.

Get written estimates for any repair work. Check credentials and contact the local Better Business Bureau or Chamber of Commerce for complaints against the businesses. Before work begins, make sure you get a written contract detailing all work to be performed, the costs, a completion day and clauses to negotiate changes and settle disputes. Also make sure the contract specifies who will get the necessary permits. Keep a copy of the signed contract.

Pay only by check or credit card.

You will be frazzled and upset and a bit desperate after a disaster, but don't let these bad people make it worse.

Bugging Out, the Hide Site and Caching

SHOULD I STAY OR SHOULD I GO?

If an evacuation has been called, such as for a hurricane, you evacuate as soon as possible.

For some situations, smart people evacuate *before* the formal announcement. For example, wild fires are unpredictable and can move fast. Better to be safe.

There is a big difference between an evacuation and bugging out.

An evacuation has the expectation that you will return to your home in the foreseeable future. In this case, it's as simple as driving away and going to your evacuation point or checking into a hotel. If you live in an area where evacuations are likely, such as a hurricane zone, plan ahead. Have a location you know you can go to and get a room or people you can stay with.

Reasons not to bug out:

You have your primary stockpile of supplies in your house.

You have a community around you who knows you and you know (this could be a good thing or a bad thing).

There is no immediate or foreseeable threat to you and your home, whether natural or man-made.

It does not appear that the situation will degrade.

When to bug out:

The most obvious would be if the home is unlivable. This would happen in the case of an extreme emergency that affects the area. Ultimately the hide site will be the place for your team to meet up if all else fails.

However, making the decision to bug out is a very difficult one if your home is still livable. Because when you bug out, there is a good probability you will not be returning to your home, so we're talking extreme emergency on a large scale.

There are several predictors on deciding to go to the hide site.

Your home is no longer livable.

The emergency or disaster is something that is approaching you and can't be stopped. The primary example of this would be a pandemic.

The rule of law has completely broken down and now your home is a target and you cannot adequately defend it

Television stations go blank.

Local FM radio stations go off the air.

The water stops.

The power grid goes down over an extensive area without any sign of repair forthcoming.

Long haul freight trucks are no longer moving. Most urban areas have enough food to last no more than a week.

You're running out of stocked supplies to the point where you're considering breaking into your main Grab-n-Go bag. Don't. Use it to get to your hide site.

Increased military presence, especially if its Federal forces, not National Guard. Federal military Army, Air Force and Marines can only be employed stateside in extreme emergencies. In your Area Study learn the difference and what National Guard units are nearby; what their unit patch is (on the left shoulder) and what unit designations would be marked on the bumpers of their military vehicles.

In cities, if garbage is piling up and not being picked up, eventually this will cause disease. It also indicates a slow breakdown of social order.

There is slim to no possibility of receiving aid. This latter is something people don't consider in mild or moderate emergencies. Localized emergencies always have the advantage of outside assistance coming in. If an emergency is on a national or international scale, this likelihood is drastically reduced.

A disturbing aspect of this is that while governments will call for evacuations, there really is no protocol for announcing that things have completely gone to s$%t. In fact, it is unlikely that such a thing will ever be announced. The desire to avoid panic will often override reality. Thus you must make this decision on your own.

Make sure you can listen in on the Emergency Broadcast Stations with your survival radio. A smart move is to monitor emergency transmissions in your area. Below is a free app that will allow you to do that. Often the emergency services are better informed than the general public. You can also get an idea of the scope of the emergency or disaster not only from what is being said, but the tone of the emergency personnel:

5-0 Police Scanner APP (Apple)	https://itunes.apple.com/us/app/5-0-radio-police-scanner/id356336433?mt=8
Fire and Police Scanner APP (Android)	https://play.google.com/store/apps/details?id=com.scannerradio&hl=en_US

THE HIDE SITE

When thinking about an hide site, use the term BLISS.

BLISS considerations for the hide site
Blends in with surrounding
Low in silhouette
Irregular in shape
Small in size
Secluded

There are, of course, exception to this guideline. There might be a time when bunkering up in a high rise might be a good option. This is if a massive chemical/biological attack makes a top floor position desirable and traveling unadvisable.

The key to the Hide Site is to stay hidden. That's your best defense. It is where you rest, recover, and live. How long depends on the emergency.

A key to the hide site is a Catch-22: water. You need water, yet water will draw other people, including predators, both human and otherwise. Consider locating the site within a half hour walk of a water source. That allows you to draw water, but not be so close that casual passerby's will stumble across your site.

The Hide Site should have concealment first and cover second. The difference between the two is this: concealment means you are hidden from observation. Cover means the position has protection against direct and indirect fire weapons (remember, arrows are indirect fire, as Custer learned). The reason I prioritize concealment over cover is because the best defense is not to be found.

The hide site is where you plan to survive during a moderate to extreme emergency when your home is untenable.

How do you get to your hide site? If you drive to it, make sure to leave the vehicle far enough away, at least two miles, so that it doesn't point others toward your site. Disable the vehicles by taking an engine part. Assume the vehicle will be looted, but perhaps you can use it if you return with the part. The easiest part to take is the main fuse or unplug the starter. You can conceal the vehicle as much as possible, but if you drove it there, it's on a trail that takes vehicles which means others can drive there too.

Another thing to consider is putting your site behind a gate that can be locked. Many parks, logging roads, etc, have lockable gates. Cut the current lock on it, drive through, out of sight, and put your own lock on the gate. Still, keep at least a two mile distance between the vehicle and your hide site.

As soon as you are settled in your site, search out an escape route and a Rally Point and make sure everyone knows where it is. The Rally Point is where you will all meet if the site is attacked.

When getting water, don't use the same trail all the time. Mix it up.

Always maintain security. One person must be up and alert at all times.

In the movie *Panic In The Year Zero*, a 1962 movie by Ray Milland, the family escapes a nuclear attack on Los Angeles towing their camper. When they get to a remote site where that had vacationed before, the father vetoes staying in the camper, over the protests of his family, and makes them move into a cave. A young couple takes over the camper, seeing it as an easy refuge. They are found shot to death within a few days. The lesson: don't take the easy location as your hide site.

Consider that others will also be running away. In an extreme emergency there will be hordes of people escaping, scavenging, and panicking. You're already better prepared than them.

Consider chokepoints and bottlenecks to your Hide Site. For example, when I lived on the Tennessee River, there were only a few bridges across it within a reasonable distance that I could take to get to the Smoky Mountains, which were a tempting location in which to plan my Hide Site. Most of those bridges were in downtown Knoxville, which meant they could easily be crowded, difficult to cross, or even shut down. Plus, the Smokies are the most visited National Park in the country with only a few roads into them—full of chokepoints. Many people would head that way in a panic.

I looked in the opposite direction, north. Oak Ridge contains vast swaths of Federal Land with no inhabitants. Not many people would think of going there (besides the glow in the dark factor). There were multiple routes to get there.

Stay away from the routes most people would naturally take, particularly Interstates. Stay away from nuclear power plants (an extended power grid down makes them unstable), military targets, and urban centers.

As soon as you are settled in your Hide Site, search out an escape route and a Rally Point and make sure everyone knows where it is. The Rally Point is where you will all meet if the Hide Site is attacked.

Always maintain security. One person must be up and alert at all times.

Some considerations.

Urban environments:

If you are in an urban environment, I recommend your Hide Site be outside of it. That means the priority is to plan how to get to it, especially considering that in high moderate and extreme emergencies, everyone will be evacuating. Do you have a route planned? One that will not be blocked?

However, take a look around. In most urban environments, there are places less traveled. Most cities are crisscrossed with an underground maze.

CACHE

Here is what to do to put in an effective cache, either at your Hide Site, or any location:

Protect the supplies. There's no point putting in a cache if when you recover it, nothing is usable. Waterproof, waterproof, waterproof. Garbage bags are not effective waterproofing. The plastic is too thin. Thick plastic should be the innermost layer. Compression sacks that seal work well. Also look at what's sold for kayakers and other who need waterproof bags. Waterproof isn't enough, though. You must also make sure the waterproof bag is protected inside of a hard case. The most common are ammunition cans. Look online and you will find commercially available hard case, waterproof containers. Large PVC pipe sealed on either end also works well.

It also does you no good to put in a cache if someone else can find it and scavenge it. Consider these variables when hiding your cache:

Disguise it. Put it in something larger that looks worthless. Can someone with a metal detector find it? Then perhaps put it inside something larger that's metal, such as a derelict car? Not in the trunk, which is where a scavenger will look.

Conceal it. The most obvious is to bury it. There is an art, however to successfully burying a cache so that it remains viable. Also, will you be able to find it again? In Special Forces we spent a large block of instruction on putting in caches. Can you bury it and then conceal the spot? How will you, or members of your team, find it and recover it?

A very effective way to cache is to sink it. Of course, it must be thoroughly waterproofed, but scavengers are very unlikely to find it. Of course, it must be in a stable place that won't get further flooded. And you must be able to recover it.

You have to put your cache in a place where others can't see you putting it or recovering it.

Consider having several smaller caches, spread out. This way, everything isn't in one place for scavengers.

What to have in your Hide Site:

The smartest supply to cache is a duplicate main Grab-n-Go bag (extreme). This accomplishes two things:

First, you have more of the essentials in all areas.

Second, if for some reason you are not able to get to your main Grab-n-Go bag, you now have one.

You can cache more supplies than a Grab-n-Go bag there. Food and extra ammunition are good ideas. Never cache a weapon.

However, the moderate cache for a hide site would contain the following:

Task Thirty-Nine
Moderate Hide Site Cache

	Emergency ration bars
	Emergency radio
	Snares
	Shelter (poncho, 550 cord)
	First Aid kit

We must be able to FIND our cache. We also might have to tell someone else how to find the cache. This means having a reference point. Pick a durable landmark that is identifiable by its title or simple description such as a bridge or stream juncture. You then locate the cache at an azimuth and distance from that point. If you get too far from this initial reference point you might then use it to go from to find a final reference point close to the cache and include specific azimuth and distance from that to the cache.

Stockpile, Scavenge, Sustain

These are the three stages of dealing with emergencies and natural disasters.

Stockpile

You've already done this doing your preparation. However, if there is an impending emergency or natural disaster, you will want to do some more.

Stockpile up to mild level initially, then move on to moderate and then extreme.

Scavenge

You will probably begin scavenging even while in the stockpile stage if the emergency or catastrophe is moderate or extreme. If you can add to your supplies, do so. Legally.

The two variables are expected length of the emergency and type.

Sustain

Sustainment occurs when it becomes clear things will not return to normal.

WHAT CAN CAUSE THE COLLAPSE OF CIVILIZATION?

World War III.

The use of nuclear, biological and chemical weapons on a large scale.

A series of local conflicts that disrupt trade and commerce on an international level.

Water shortages. This is one of the most glaring threats to our world. Many places in the world already lack clean water. I predict that wars in the future will not be over oil, but over water.

Climate change. While people debate this, I prefer to deal with the scientific reality that we are damaging our environment and Mother Nature has a way of equalizing things.

A large solar flare that bathes the planet in an EMP pulse that destroys electronics.

A pandemic. One *will* happen and sooner, rather than later.

Over-population, which leads to a depletion of resources.

Zombies. Which actually is a form of pandemic.

A meteor strike of sufficient size.

A volcanic eruption that spreads enough ash to start the equivalent of a nuclear winter.

Economic disruption that spreads.

Remember that great civilizations have collapsed before. Often it wasn't a single event, but an accumulation of events. The Mayans, Mesopotamia, Persia, Greece, Rome, and on and on. While I am not an alarmist, I think we have a reasonably good chance of seeing a major disruption of our way of life in the next thirty years. As they used to say in the old Army, when they had cigarettes in the C-Rations: Smoke 'em if you got 'em.

Less than that, there are a number of various possibilities. What most people fail to realize is how fragile civilization is and how easily it can break down, with a domino effect that will be shocking.

In researching this, I found many of those addressing this issue are either naïve or gloss over the depth of what will happen. Many dwell on political issues. I'm just going to focus on the practical issues.

While New York and New Jersey struggled to recover from Hurricane Sandy, a friend emailed that they got their power back, and a crew from Alabama had been working in their neighborhood day and night doing this. While this shows the great spirit of America, it occurs to me that that crew would not be there is Alabama needed them. This is key: a large-scale catastrophe that covers most of a continent will preclude aid from inside that continent.

Pre-Collapse

There are stages to surviving an extreme emergency. While a dramatic event might bring it about, it is more likely you will see many signs indicating the collapse is coming. Most people will ignore these signs. The closest I can liken it to is Germany in the 1930s. Many people saw what was coming; the vast majority chose to ignore it. On a much lower level, as the housing market bubbled and boiled in 2006, my wife and I sold our house, against the advice of pretty much everyone. We crunched the numbers and also accepted that things *had* to change, and not in a good way.

You will see signs of bad things coming. It won't happen overnight. Severe power outages that don't get better are another sign.

The key to pre-collapse is, like everything in this book, to prepare. The base level of survival, Grab & Go bags, etc. will not be sufficient. Some preparations can be integrated into your current life as a way of living, such as growing a garden. But you have to start *now*.

I'm not going to cover the likelihood of various scenarios, because it's just as likely a random, unexpected event can cause the collapse of civilization as easily as war, peak oil, global warming, etc etc.

The bottom line is it isn't going to be pretty. You can expect food shortages, fuel shortages, riots, power outages, martial law, war and the complete breakdown of law and order.

And that's only the first month.

I cannot overemphasize how quickly the veneer of civilization can be stripped away. Some of the ethnic fighting in various places around the world have shown how quickly apparently civilized people can rapidly fall into barbarism. In 10th Special Forces, I found many of our soldiers were most dismayed by the fighting they saw in the Balkans because those places seemed so much like their own home (Sarajevo hosted the Olympics not long before the war). We tend to think this 'can't happen here' but it can.

Another key to wrap your brain around is that there won't be any help coming. Once civilization breaks down, there won't be a reaching out from any remaining pockets. They will be desperate for their own survival. Supermarkets have a three-day supply of food. The world, the entire world, has about a month and a half supply. One of the signs will be panic buying. You don't want to be caught up in the panic.

On the plus side, you will be amazed how quickly many human beings can adapt to a change in their standard of living. While we will miss our cell phones and lights and supermarkets, we can adapt and evolve.

An extreme emergency requires an extreme mindset. You have to let go of many habits.

So what do you need to do to prepare?

Prioritize your needs based on your area study. The first question is if you can even stay where you are. If you are in a metropolitan area, most likely not. If you live in the suburbs, consider that you will see massive urban flight through your communities. Where can you go? This is taking the concept of the hide site to a whole new level. Since you have now done all your preparations for mild and moderate emergencies it's time to take it to the next level and prepare for an extreme emergency.

The priorities are the same except on a *sustainable*, long-term basis: water, food, shelter.

The key word is sustainable. You can stock up a year's worth of food and have a water source, but that's not sustainable. Also, a food stock, like any other, is subject to being taken from you.

Here's a sobering thought: few areas in the United States are locally self-sustaining. Without industrialized food processing, we simply can't produce enough food to feed our current population level. Think what that means: many people will starve to death. Starving people are desperate people and they will do anything to get food. So your food stock will be like fresh brains to zombies.

Can you live off the land? Do you know how? Do you want to learn how to?

There are things you can stock up on that will be useful. While initially, cash and valuables such as gold coins might have value, when things get desperate enough, other items will become more precious. Weapons and ammunition are two of those. Medical supplies are another. So is food. So is expertise, especially medical.

I'm not going to rehash what's already been covered in equipment. Look at what has been discussed and then consider it in terms of years of use.

Collapse
Run for the hills boys!

Not necessarily. Evaluate the situation. If you are not in immediate danger, this is a moment when taking your time is important. Gather as much information as possible, understanding that you will hear conflicting accounts. There will be an effort by those in power to suppress panic. Remember reading or hearing about the original broadcast of *War of the Worlds*?

There were those on 9-11 who evacuated the second tower, and then went back to their offices when given the all clear. I've listened to tapes of some of those people on their cell phones, decrying this decision as they were trapped after the second plane hit. Be very leery of those who declare an emergency over. In many emergency situations there are after-effects, whether it be follow-on earthquakes, more bombs set for first responders in a terrorist attack, or others.

How do you know civilization has collapsed? When the infrastructure (electricity, roads, rail, flight) fails and does not appear to be coming back any time soon. Many people will wait for help. Unfortunately, the help will be in the same situation. It's a question of considering your hide site your new home, or, if untenable, moving until you find a locale where you can develop a self-sustaining community for your team.

Speed of Collapse

Understand that a collapse can be a gradual thing or it can happen very quickly. There are some keys that collapse is imminent. Steer away from the fear mongers who warn you that society is going to collapse and you should run out and invest in gold or whatever product they're hawking. Their goal is to make money, which makes little sense if they truly believe society is collapsing. My theory is that it is a possibility, but not a probability.

More signs of the fall:

- Power outages that cover entire regions and show little sign of being restored.
- Multiple nuclear explosions.
- A solar flare that fries the world's electrical grid.
- When an endemic (confined to a particular area) becomes a pandemic (spread over all areas). A pandemic also has a higher infection rate and usually a higher kill rate.
- Remember, a huge problem you will face is that most people, unlike you, are *not* prepared for emergencies. Panic is inevitable regardless of the emergency, especially if it affects everyone in your area.

SCAVENGE

Consider this stage two ways. The most obvious is when you have to do the scavenging. But there is also the danger of those who try to scavenge you and your stockpile, since you are already prepared.

Defense against scavenging: Here are keys:

Be aware of your situation. What are current threats, growing threats and potential threats?

Avoid conflict if at all possible.

Are you armed? Are you willing to use your weapons?

Make your situation a hard target. Simple scavengers go for the easiest targets first. How many people know you have stockpiled supplies? This is not something you want to broadcast. If they know, do they know you are also prepared to defend your supplies?

Act decisively. This is something you should have done during your Area Study. How far are you willing to go to defend your home and when will you bug out? You will go even further to defend your hide site, because you wouldn't be in them if it wasn't a high moderate to extreme emergency.

Be prepared to retreat. You defend up to a point, but discretion is smarter than being overwhelmed. Part of bugging out of your home is when you know it is no longer defendable. You have designated your Rally Point and kept your Grab-n-Go bag packed. In the face of overwhelming attack, retreat.

Your first choice is to scare scavengers off. Your second is to retreat. Your last option is to incapacitate scavengers. If you go to this mode it's all or nothing.

A sad reality of extreme situations is that the bad people will be more decisive and act more ruthlessly than the good people.

You want to be the alive people.

There is a line between scavenging and looting. That lines moves as the situation becomes more extreme. In a life and death situation, there is no line.

People will loot if given the opportunity. A power outage in an urban environment is one such opportunity. During this, your goal is stay secure. Looters are not looking for things they need to survive. They're simply criminals taking advantage of the situation.

The timeline on when people turn into scavenger depends, but during Hurricane Katrina, things deteriorated after only 48 hours.

Legitimate scavengers take only what they need for survival. However, scavenging other people in a survival situation is criminal and unethical. You scavenge places, not people.

Where to Scavenge

This is only limited by your imagination and location. As with every topic, there are so many variables, so there are no hard and fast rules.

A major consideration is to accept that if you are in scavenge mode, so are others. Less prepared people will actually go into this mode *before* you do. Thus, they will be more experienced. They will also be more desperate.

Be counter-intuitive. Don't go for the obvious.

Where to scavenge will be determined by what supplies you need in priority order. How much you scavenge depends on how desperate your situation is.

This is something you should have considered during your Area Study. Take a look at your map. What's in the area? Housing, factories, parks, businesses, hospitals, schools, etc.?

The following is a list of locations, along with what can be found there. Note that some places will yield supplies you might not expect to find there.

Houses. Make sure any home you scavenge isn't occupied. It's not worth fighting over. You'll search depending on your needs. Meds? Food? Clothing? Don't forget the attic, basement and garage. Garages can yield surprising results. Consider sustainment items such as seeds and gardening tools. Trash bags for waterproofing and carrying your supplies. Something that people will miss are water filters! A high end home might have very effective filters that you can rip out and use at your hide site. Coffee filters are also useful to clean water before having to boil it. View the house as you did when you were looking at your own house for survival. There is drinkable water in the same places—the water heater for example.

Apartment buildings. More bang to time than single houses as they hold multiple homes. Don't forget the parking garage where you can search . . .

Cars and trucks. If you are mobile in your own vehicle you can scavenge gas and parts. However, vehicles can yield other supplies such as food, weapons, and water. Check the glove compartment. Check the trunk. Tire iron? Emergency kit? A car jack that can used to get into other places? Check the engine. Do you need the wiring? Does the battery still have life? Tires can be burned to make an emergency signal with black smoke. NEVER use gas to start a fire. Mirrors can be used for signaling. Abandoned semi-trucks can be full of whatever!

ATV and Off-Road shop. ATVs are a better form of transportation than cars in severe emergencies. Remember, vehicles require . . .

Gas stations. The obvious goal here is gas, although getting it out of the ground tanks without power requires you have to have a pump (battery or hand powered) and a long enough siphon hose. There are easier ways to get gas.

Automotive stores. For vehicle parts.

Food and grocery stores. These will be first targets of scavengers and will quickly be picked clean. Don't forget to check in the back, where the restock is stored. You might consider *avoiding* these places in the early stages of an extreme emergency. After all, you have your own stockpile. Perhaps bypass the stores and go to the . . .

Distribution Center. During your Area Study, did you find local and regional distribution centers for stores? These will be full of supplies and not initially be on most people's scavenging radar as they go for the low hanging fruit first. Don't forget to check the semi-trailers parked outside that might not have been unloaded or recently loaded.

Restaurants. Food, but also check for knives, pots and pans.

Bars. You really don't need alcohol, but check for bottled water. Weapons hidden under and behind the bar.

Schools (including colleges and community colleges). First aid kits. Tools in the maintenance room. Does it have a shop class?

Hospitals. What are you priorities medically? Again, though, these will be among the first targets for scavengers. Also, they will be a place people will congregate. Depending on the threat, it might also harbor the threat, such as a pandemic.

Pharmacies. Initially people will go for the drugs. There are other items that might be overlooked. Ace wraps are very useful for a variety of things. Bandages. While most people think of hospitals and pharmacies first for medical supplies, consider these . . .

Veterinarians and animal hospitals. These are stocked with medical supplies, including medications

Nursing homes. Ditto.

Storage units. It's certain some people have put their emergency stash in a locked storage unit. In addition, there are all sorts of supplies to be found, concentrated in one place.

Office buildings. Often they will have first aid kits and some emergency gear in them. Consider what kind of business it was. What will be there? Check desk drawers.

Police stations. Weapons. Tools. Emergency kits. Radios. The Terminator.

Churches: Check the basement and offices. Many conduct food drives and have kitchens.

Fire stations. First aid kits, emergency tools, radios. A pump truck could hold hundreds of gallons of water. Don't assume its potable.

Military posts and National Guard Armories. If abandoned, they might contain weapons and other equipment. However, to get to a level where you're scavenging, the National Guard and military were most likely already called out and deployed.

Animal Control Centers. Guess where you can find traps?

Dumpsters. One man's trash is another man's treasure. They can also be shelters.

Dumps. You never know.

Train stations. Vending machines, restaurants. Check the bathrooms. The lockers.

Trains. Check the luggage.

Airports. There are supplies inside an airport and restaurants and stores. Also, think of the parking lots, rich with all those vehicles. And gas in those cars.

Aircraft. Check the galley. The luggage.

Pawn Shops. Full of interesting things, especially firearms.

Pet Stores. Lots of food.

Marinas. Check not only the marina, but abandoned boats. A boat can be an excellent base camp, depending on the threat, where you are, and if you know what you're doing.

Farms. Look not only at the house and the barn, but what's being grown. Could it be a source of sustainable food?

Libraries and bookstores. This is a place that almost all scavengers will bypass or ignore, but is the most important if you are in scavenge mode. Because it is possible you will transition from scavenge mode into sustain mode, rather than recovery. Books are knowledge. Knowledge is power. You have this book. Get others that are on topics you need and will need. Get books that will help you transition into sustainment. How to farm. How to make things.

How to Scavenge

When on the move in an emergency or catastrophe, you should always be on the lookout for useful materials as needed. Don't hoard, but complement what you already have. Also, save your stockpile of prepared material as much as possible by using scavenged supplies.

If you are in your home or hide site and need supplies, you must plan a scavenging expedition. This not something to be done lightly. If you are in scavenge mode, so are others. And you are all looking for the same supplies.

That's the first planning consideration. What are the priorities of supplies needed? You don't simply list everything you need. You prioritize. People can only carry so much, but you might also have your scavenging time cut short by the presence of others.

After you have determined the scavenging objective (location and priorities of supplies), the first step is to send a scout. The scout should have optics and a way to communicate back. It is optimal to put 24 hours of surveillance on any target because you then have an entire daily cycle of observation. The scout must have a communication schedule to strictly follow and a time limit to return. If either of those two pass, you must consider the scout compromised, along with your location.

The scout should check the objective for ingress and egress. Dangers. Special equipment that will be needed, such as bolt cutters. Whether the objective is damaged and dangerous structurally.

Once the scout reports back, it's time to put together the expedition. Never send someone alone. Always work in at least buddy teams. Someone is designated as the leader. Factors include how much is needed and how much can be carried. Plan security on the move and at the objective. Everyone should carry:

Tools for scavenging:
Gloves.
Mask.
Flashlight.
Multi-tool.
Bolt cutters.
A backpack. As many empty bags as they can carry when full. Also remember, you can scavenge a location and then spend time moving material out and caching it nearby where other scavengers wouldn't look. Then go back for it. Also consider things like a wheel barrow, a bike with baskets, etc. to carry supplies.

Everyone should have gloves, multitool, flashlight, and weapon. The expedition should have at least one crowbar. If you are scavenging gas, you need a siphon and containers.

The scavenging party must have a Rally Point where they will regroup if attacked or forced to disperse while on the expedition. This Rally Point is *not* simply going back to the home/hide site. In fact, it should be in a direction that will not lead others to the home/hide site.

If going into a large building, you must have a way to mark your way back out. Glow sticks, spray paint, markers. Remember, any mark you leave tells other you exist and were there.

Scavenging is only limited by your imagination, your resources, your environment and the type of emergency/catastrophe.

In Conclusion

What you need above all a *determination to survive.* All else is secondary. Even if things look hopeless, you can't ever give up.

You're capable of what is unimaginable to you right now.

In Special Forces we found a *sense of humor* could make the most difficult situation look a little brighter. In my team Standing Operating Procedures, under my commander's policy letter, the last thing listed was to "keep your sense of humor, you're going to need it." Laughter can be a pressure release. That's the reason why I put some in this book. When we take ourselves too seriously, we lose track of the purpose of surviving.

As part of that, you also need to be able to *let it go.* Don't dwell on bad luck, past mistakes, or losses. Negative thinking drains energy. Deal with the present, prepare for the future and accept you can't change the past.

But you also can't control everything in the future either. You have to face it with a positive attitude but also accept that the *future is uncertain.* This entire book is based on that fact. It would be great if your current situation continues and you never face an emergency or survival situation or accident or disaster, but you have no guarantees. One symptom of disaster situations is that there will be considerable confusion and disinformation initially. Both because it won't be clear what's going on, but also factor in people spreading false information to further their own ends or sprouting from their fear and panic. You have to sort through it all and make the best possible decisions.

We're in this together.

In conclusion, you will find that the traits of the survivor are also the traits, in everyday, normal living, make a person successful. So you can use this book not only to prepare, but also to learn traits that will make your current environment more fruitful and positive.

THE END

Author's Note: since things are constantly changing, please email if you find outdated links. Also, please send comments, suggestions, etc. to
bob@bobmayer.com

Additionally, I run workshops on preparing the Area Study. If interested, please contact me.
I have numerous free, downloadable slideshows about survival and other topics. Go to
www.bobmayer.com/workshops

Thanks for the read!
If you enjoyed the book, please leave a review.
Cool Gus likes them as much as he likes squirrels!

If you want some intriguing reads about a couple of great disasters we can learn from, excerpts from my two books: **Stuff Doesn't Just Happen: The Gift of Failure** are available. They are the story of the St. Francis Dam failure, one of the greatest engineering disasters in the 20th Century and The Donner Party, a look inside the poor planning and decision making that led to that event. They are on my Freebies page.
http://bobmayer.com/freebies/
Additionally, Who Dares Wins: Special Operations Strategies for Success is available on all eBook platforms via
http://bobmayer.com/nonfiction/

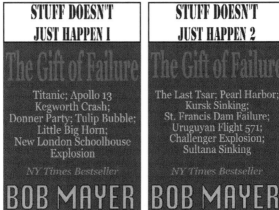

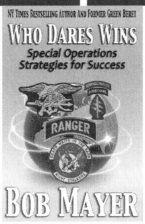

About the Author

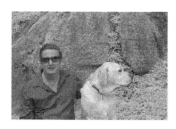

Look! Squirrel!
Bob is a NY Times Bestselling author, graduate of
West Point, former Green Beret and the feeder of Cool
Gus. He's had over 75 books published including the
#1 series Area 51, Atlantis, Time Patrol and The Green
Berets. Born in the Bronx, having traveled the world
(usually not tourist spots), he now lives peacefully
with his wife and lab.

For information on all his books, please get a free
copy of the **_Reader's Guide_**. You can download it in
mobi (Amazon) ePub (iBooks, Nook, Kobo) or PDF,
from his home page at www.bobmayer.com

**For free eBooks, short stories and audio short
stories, please go to** http://bobmayer.com/freebies/
The page includes free and discounted book
constantly updated.
Permanently free:
Eyes of the Hammer (Green Beret series book #1)
Duty (Duty, Honor, Country series book #1)

Ides of March (Time Patrol)
There are also free shorts stories and free
audiobook stories.

There are over 220 free, downloadable
Powerpoint presentations via Slideshare on a wide
range of topics from history, to survival, to writing, to
book trailers. This page and slideshows are constantly
updated at:
http://bobmayer.com/workshops/

If you're interested in audiobooks, you can
download one for free and test it out here: Audible

Questions, comments, suggestions:
Bob@BobMayer.com
Blog: http://bobmayer.com/blog/
Twitter: https://twitter.com/Bob_Mayer
Facebook:
https://www.facebook.com/authorbobmayer
Google +:
https://plus.google.com/u/0/101425129105653262
515
Instagram:
https://www.instagram.com/sifiauthor/
Youtube:
https://www.youtube.com/user/IWhoDaresWins
Subscribe to his newsletter for the latest news,
free eBooks, audio, etc.

Appendix A: All Tasks/Checklists

Task One
Mild: Get two cases of bottled water for each person in your household.

Task Two
Mild: A-Team Contact Information & Alert Flow

A-Team Member	*Cell Phone Number*	*Work/School Address & Phone #*
#1		
#2		
#3		
#4		
#5		
#6		
#7		
#8		
#9		
#10		

Mild: Out of Area Contact, Immediate Rally Point, Emergency Rally Point

Out of area contact location, phone #	
Immediate Rally Point location	
Emergency Rally Point location	

Mild: Emergency Information

Place	Phone	Address
Poison Control	**800-222-1222**	N/A
Work #1 for ?		
Work #2 for ?		
School #1 for ?		
School #2 for ?		
Closest police station		
Closest emergency room		
Closest fire station		
Power company/ Gas company		
Water company		
Family Doctor		
Health Insurance & Account #		
Insurance company Account #		

Task Three
Mild: If you don't have one, get a first aid kit for your home.

Example:
First Aid kit: Adventure Med Kit Weekender:
http://amzn.to/2f3gh4c

Task Four
Mild: Evaluate & list the following for you and each member of your A-Team.

Name:	
Ability to react in an Emergency:	
Special Skill/Background #1:	
Special Skill/Background #2:	
Special Skill/Background #3:	
Special Skill/Background #4	

Task Five
Mild: Evaluate and list the following for you and each member of your A-Team.

Name:	
Overall physical condition:	
Medical status:	
Allergies:	
Medications:	
Ability to walk/run:	
Special needs:	
Able to swim?	
Able to drive? Access to a vehicles?	

Task Six
Mild: Fall Prevention Checklist

	Item	
	Clear clutter	
	Secure edges of all rugs	
	Secure rugs to floors so they don't bunch or slide	
	Place grab bars and non-slip mats in bathrooms	
	Make sure all stairways and dark areas are adequately lit AMIR motion sensor light: https://amzn.to/2LwlkKY	
	Wear slippers or shows with rubber bottoms at all time—no socks only!	
	Childproof stairs with gates at top and bottom	
	Do all stairs have handrails?	
	Use ladders properly according to specifications	

Task Seven
Mild: Poison Prevention Checklist

	Post Poison Control Number prominently in Kitchen 800-222-1222	
	Label all unmarked liquid containers	
	Insure all cleaning products are stored out of reach of children	
	Insure all medications are stored out of reach of children	
	Put childproof locks on all reachable cabinets	
	Never mix household cleaning products	
	Never mix medications without approval	
	Monitor all heaters and fireplaces for CO2	
	Have fireplaces cleaned annually	

Task Eight
Mild: Choking/Suffocation Prevention Checklist

	Keep small toys, items out of reach of toddlers	
	Clear sleeping areas for babies from all possible items that could smother them	
	Keep trash bags and plastic bags out of reach of children	
	Keep batteries, especially button batteries, from children	

Task Nine. Mild: Drowning Prevention Checklist

	Never leave water running when not being watched	
	Always monitor small children while bathing	
	Don't use electronics around water, especially bathtub	
	Keep toilet lids closed	
	Pool must be enclosed by minimum 4 foot high fence with childproof gate	
	Never allow children to swim unsupervised	

Task Ten
Mild: Fire Prevention Checklist

	Smoke detectors in every bedroom	
	Smoke detector on every floor	
	Test smoke detectors every money	
	Replace smoke detector batteries every six months	
	Never leave kitchen while stove is on	
	Never leave candles burning overnight or when not home	

Task Eleven
Mild: Firearm Prevention Checklist

	All firearms must be secured in a locked area	
	Locked trigger guards on all firearms	
	Never leave a loaded firearm unattended	
	Know and follow all firearm safety rules	

Task Twelve

Go to Homefacts http://www.homefacts.com/ and enter your zip code.

Task Thirteen
Mild: Of the four type of special environments, which ones do you need to be concerned with in order of priority: Cold Weather, Desert, Tropical and Water.

Special Environments
1.
2.
3.

Natural Disasters in Order of Likelihood
1.
2.
3.

Task Fourteen. Mild: Man-made disasters in order of likelihood in your AO

1.	
2.	
3.	
4.	
5.	

Task Fifteen. Mild: GPS/Map Checklist

	Road atlas for each car. Rand McNally Road Atlas. https://amzn.to/2LwlO3B	
	Download or buy topographic maps for your area of operation: National Geographic Maps: http://www.natgeomaps.com/trail-maps/pdf-quads USGS Maps: http://nationalmap.gov/ustopo/	
	Get a waterproof map case to put your top maps in, with dummy cord. Waterproof map case. https://amzn.to/2BBhaNm	
	Get a topographic atlas of your area. DeLorme Tennessee Atlas: https://amzn.to/2BBhwna	
	Download the map tiles for your area of operation for your car GPS (if possible), your phone, and handheld GPS (if used)	

Task Sixteen
Mild: Download Locator Apps

Road ID Here is their home page with links to both Apple and Android along with information on how the app works. https://www.roadid.com/pages/road-id-app	
Life 360 Android: https://play.google.com/store/apps/details?id=com.life360.android.safetymapd Apple: https://itunes.apple.com/us/app/life360-family-tracker/id384830320?mt=8	
Sygic Family locator Android: https://play.google.com/store/apps/details?id=com.sygic.familywhere.android&hl=cs&referrer=utm_source%3Dsygic-com%26utm_medium%3Dheader-features%26utm_campaign%3Dfamily-locator Apple: https://itunes.apple.com/sk/app/family-locator-gps-tracker/id588364107?mt=8	
Trusted Contacts: Android: https://play.google.com/store/apps/details?id=com.google.android.apps.emergencyassist&utm_source=google&utm_medium=web&utm_campaign=homepage Apple: https://itunes.apple.com/app/trusted-contacts/id1225684042	

Task Seventeen
Mod/Ex: A-Team Code Word List

Word/Phrase	Code Word
Home	
IRP	
ERP	
HIDE SITE	
I've been compromised and am sending this under duress.	
Code name for team member #1:	
Code name for team member #2:	
Code name for team member #3:	
Code name for team member #4:	
Code name for team member #5:	
Code name for team member #6:	
Code word for every day of week.	
Anchor Point for team	
Add whatever key words you believe you need	

Task Eighteen
Mild: If you don't have one, get an emergency radio for your home.

Example:
Survival radio: https://amzn.to/2BBBaiN

Task Nineteen
Mild: Water Checklist

Completed		Expiration date
	3 gallons of water per person 2 cases	Rotate every six months
	2 bottles of water in car.	Rotate every six months
	2 bottles of water in work/school GnG bag	Rotate every six months

Task Twenty
Mod/Ex: Water Checklist

		Expiration date
	Moderate: 3 gallons of water per person 2 cases	Rotate every six months
	Moderate: Portable water filter. Katadyn Water Microfilter: https://amzn.to/2LBYcuE	Expiration date of cartridge
	Extreme: 30 gallons per person or more (10 cases, 55 gallon drum, etc)	Rotate every six months
	Mod/Ex: location of drinkable water source near home	Make sure it is safe
	Mod/Ex: GnG Bag: bottle of water purifying pills	Expiration date on bottle
	Mod/Ex GnG bag: Survival Straw LifeStraw Personal Water Filter: https://amzn.to/2V4uUJf	
	Mod/Ex: One case of water in car.	Rotate every six months
	Extreme: BOHS—drinkable water source near hide site.	Make sure it is safe

Task Twenty-One
Mild: Rotation and Inspection Checklist

Rotate or Check Every:	Item
Month. (1st of each month)	Test fire alarms
Quarterly (1 Jan, 1 April, 1 July, 1 Oct)	Gas in spare cans, Power bars, emergency water in vehicle,
Semi-Annual (1 Jan, 1 July)	Replace fire alarm batteries; check first aid kits
Annual (1 Jan)	Gng bags

Task Twenty-Two
Mild: Food Checklist

Completed		Expiration date
	3 days of non-perishable food. 2,400 calories per day per person	Rotate as needed
	Non-electric can opener	
	Power Bars: https://amzn.to/2Rd54DN	Check Expiration date

Task Twenty-Three
Mod/Ex: Food Checklist

Completed		Expiration
	Moderate: A week's worth of non-perishable food. 2,400 calories per day per person	
	Extreme: A month's worth of non-perishable food. 2,400 calories per day per person Mountain House Essential Bucket: https://amzn.to/2BAkM21	
	Mod/Ex: Emergency Rations Grizzly Gear: https://amzn.to/2Lzqk1l ERbar: https://amzn.to/2SfllW4 DaTrex 3600: https://amzn.to/2LzqtBV	Check Expiration date
	Mod/Ex: A means of cooking food away from home. MSR Dragon Fly: https://amzn.to/2SgoTHz	Rotate as needed
	Mod/Ex: Scavenging, hunting and gathering. Covered under Survival.	
	Multivitamins: Two months worth	

Task Twenty-Four. Mild: First Aid Checklist

	First Aid kit: Adventure Med Kit Weekender: http://amzn.to/2f3gh4c	
	Quikclot sponge: http://amzn.to/2fkHgMr	
	Red Cross First Aid App (Apple): https://itunes.apple.com/us/app/first-aid-by-american-red/id529160691?mt=8 (Android): https://play.google.com/store/apps/details?id=com.cube.arc.fa&hl=en	
	iTriage App (Apple): https://itunes.apple.com/us/app/itriage-symptom-checker/id304696939 (Android): https://play.google.com/store/apps/details?id=com.healthagen.iTriage	
	CPR and choking app: (Apple): https://itunes.apple.com/app/cpr-choking/id314907949 **CPR and Choking (Android):** https://play.google.com/store/apps/details?id=org.learncpr.videoapp	
	Medical Alert Badges as needed	
	Annual Physical	
	Glasses as backup if use contacts--Extra pair of glasses	
	1 week supply of medications	
	Car: First Aid kit: Adventure Med Kit Weekender: http://amzn.to/2f3gh4c	

Task Twenty-Five
Mod/Ex: First Aid Checklist

Completed		
	First Aid Kit: Lifeline 4038 Hard Shell: http://amzn.to/2eSbS3H	
	Trauma Pack w/ Quik-Clot https://amzn.to/2Rbyxy0	
	Universal Splint, rolled: http://amzn.to/2f3eCfe	
	Recon Tourniquet: https://amzn.to/2Lzt1jt	
	Complete a CPR course	
	Complete a First Aid Course	
	1 month of medications; know homeopathic replacements	
	GnG bag: First Aid kit: Adventure Med Kit Weekender: http://amzn.to/2f3gh4c	

Task Twenty-Six. Mild: Shelter Checklist

	Walking boots/shoes at work/school/car with socks	
	Proper clothing for your environment	
	Gloves, hat	
	Car: rain jacket or poncho	
	Car: Blanket	

Task Twenty-Seven. Mod/Ex Shelter Checklist

Walking boots/shoes at work/school/car with socks	
Proper outdoor clothing for your environment	
Watch cap and/or boonie hat: Watch cap: https://amzn.to/2LvL5uX Boonie Hat: https://amzn.to/2QKgI9X	
Car: rain jacket or poncho Rain jacket: Poncho: https://amzn.to/2LvsWx8	
Car: Blanket and Emergency Bivy sack: https://amzn.to/2R7FLmP	

Task Twenty-Eight. Mild: Fire Checklist

	Fire extinguisher in kitchen	
	Fire extinguisher in each floor and near fireplaces	
	Fire extinguisher in car	
	Study fire drill safety in Survival portion and share with household	
	Fire drill in household every six months	
	Designate IRP in case of fire	
	Emergency ladder in all bedrooms above the first floor sufficient to reach the ground from a window. First Alert 2-Story Escape Ladder: https://amzn.to/2V65M4Z First Alert 3-Story Escape Ladder: https://amzn.to/2SdhatX	

Task Twenty-Nine
Mod/Ex : Fire Checklist

	A means of cooking meals in home if power is out.
	Storm proof lighters (least 1 each home, GnG, car) **Storm proof lighters:** **https://amzn.to/2Cv8yt7**
	Storm proof matches (1 ea GnG, home): **https://amzn.to/2V5tEWe**
	Portable Stove (same as Food, Mod/Ex) **MSR Dragon Fly:** **https://amzn.to/2SgoTHz**
	Extreme: Learn how to start a fire with items found in nature

Task Thirty. Mild: Scan and store in cloud and on thumb drive the following documents.
Then put in a mobile, fireproof secure box

Stored	Scanned	Cloud	Documents
			Birth Certificates
			Passports/Visas
			Home insurance documents
			Car insurance documents and registration
			Health insurance documents/Medical Cards
			Employment records
			Tax returns
			Drivers licenses
			Social Security Card
			Back-up ID (student ID, military, VA, etc.)
			Credit Cards
			Medical history
			Power of attorney
			Wills
			Concealed carry license
			Important phone numbers
			Titles/Deeds/etc
			Marriage License
			Financial accounts with account #, phone #, address,
			All military and VA records
			Thumb drive with video of house and all contents

Task Thirty-One. Mild: Emergency equipment checklist for work/school

	Item
	Battery operated emergency radio and/or TV
	Non-perishable 3 day supply of food for each person
	Bottled water for 3 days for each employee (2 cases per)
	Blankets, pillows, cots
	First aid kits
	First aid manual
	Flashlights, batteries, light sticks
	Toolkit
	Whistle, flare, to signal for help
	VS-17 or similar panel to signal for help, especially if forced to roof
	A designated IRP for all personnel outside the building
	Tarps, heavy duty plastic trash bags and duct tape
	Everyone knows building evacuation routes
	Emergency drills at least every six months/as required by law

Task Thirty-Two. Mild: Car equipment checklist

	Pre-packaged Roadside emergency kit (show below with list of items) https://amzn.to/2CylcaV This contains some of the items below—full list follows.
	2 bottles of water
	Fire extinguisher: https://amzn.to/2V4u8fz
	Driver's license, proof of insurance, insurance company contact number
	Cell phone charger cable
	First Aid kit: Adventure Med Kit Weekender: http://amzn.to/2f3gh4c
	Reflective warning triangles: https://amzn.to/2SknVKE
	Flashlight with red warning flasher
	Blanket and Emergency bivy sack: https://amzn.to/2R7FLmP
	Life Hammer: https://amzn.to/2A8HL4r
	Ice scraper
	Work gloves
	Flat tire inflation canister: https://amzn.to/2CvN7s6
	Road maps as already designated under GPS/Maps
	Walking shoes/boots and socks as already designated
	Keychain pill fob with extra medication: https://amzn.to/2V9spoX

Task Thirty-Three. Mod/Ex: Car equipment checklist

	Case of water or the equivalent (minimum 3 gallons)
	Collapsible Snow Shovel (based on Area Study)https://amzn.to/2rWOKc9
	Toolkit
	Jumper cables
	GoTreads Emergency Traction: https://amzn.to/2ShCnCV
	Tow straps
	Poncho: https://amzn.to/2LvsWx8
	Road side flares (I prefer battery power lights): https://amzn.to/2CF8nvt
	Spare fuses for your vehicle
	Spare bulbs for turn signals and brake lights for your vehicle
	Extra quart of oil
	Duct tape
	Battery powered siphon: https://amzn.to/2SegtAI
	Multipurpose tool: https://amzn.to/2Lzt3bh and/or Leatherman Crunch tool: https://amzn.to/2BD3lxR
	Emergency Battery Charger: https://amzn.to/2LwEu3p
	Survival radio: https://amzn.to/2BBBaiN

Task Thirty-Four. Mild: Travel checklist

	Passport and copy of your passport. Scan your passport and upload it to the cloud
	Health insurance card
	Extra credit card carried separate from your wallet/purse along with copy of passport
	Written list of emergency contact numbers (in case you lose your cell phone)
	Prepaid long distance calling card
	A few blank checks if you don't normally carry your check book
	Medication plus at least 3 extra days than the trip is planned
	Protein bars
	Cash

Task Thirty-Five. Mild: Personal Items checklist

	Leatherman: https://amzn.to/2Cxvyry
	AAA flashlight in case with Leatherman
	Cell phone
	Credit Card Survival Tool: https://amzn.to/2CvDOYX

Task Thirty-Six
Mod/Ex: Survival Vest checklist

	Vest: https://amzn.to/2Cxvyry
	Israeli Battle Dressings: https://amzn.to/2LzJSm6
	Quikclot gauze: https://amzn.to/2BHIdXs
	Storm proof lighters: https://amzn.to/2BBC4Md
	Survival Knife: https://amzn.to/2LwgGfQ
	Compass: https://amzn.to/2GAOycI
	Map and case. Already covered.
	Assorted zip ties along with Handcuff zip ties: https://amzn.to/2Rdar61

Task Thirty-Seven
Mild: Grab-n-Go checklist

	First aid kit: https://amzn.to/2RdEc6Q
	Emergency Radio: https://amzn.to/2GCTMEJ
	Hand crank Flashlight: https://amzn.to/2Vg1bgK
	Emergency rations—one of the following Grizzly Gear: https://amzn.to/2Lzqk1l ERbar: https://amzn.to/2SfllW4 DaTrex 3600: https://amzn.to/2LzqtBV
	Poncho: https://amzn.to/2CxAY5G
	Water 6 bottles
	550/parachute cord: https://amzn.to/2CxSneD
	Extra keys home/car
	Extra medication
	Extra set of glasses
	Boots/workout shoes/socks

Task Thirty-Eight. Mod/Ex Grab-n-Go checklist

	WATER
	4 water bottles
	Water containers/canteens/Camelbak
	Lifestraw: https://amzn.to/2V8udyM
	Water filter: https://amzn.to/2V7PIjb
	Water purifying tablets: https://amzn.to/2LAqndh
	Waterproof sacks
	Compressible water containers: https://amzn.to/2Lzj1qC
	FIRE
	Stormproof lighters: https://amzn.to/2V8Ld87
	Windproof matches: https://amzn.to/2SkR2x9
	Magnesium fire starter: https://amzn.to/2SjWkJk
	Portable stove and fuel: https://amzn.to/2Lzj59Q
	FOOD
	3 day supply food
	Emergency rations Grizzly Gear: https://amzn.to/2Lzqk1l **ERbar:** https://amzn.to/2SfllW4 **DaTrex 3600:** https://amzn.to/2LzqtBV

Cooking pots: https://amzn.to/2SenkKs **Utensils:** https://amzn.to/2Afz0p7
FIRST AID
First aid kit: https://amzn.to/2RdEc6Q
Quikclot bandage, First Aid bandage, rolled splint: https://amzn.to/2VbgcAb
Extra medication for one week at least
Extra glasses (old pair is better than nothing)
SHELTER
Emergency bivy sack: https://amzn.to/2BDuPDx
Small tent or poncho
550/parachute cord: https://amzn.to/2CxSneD
Tent stakes if just using poncho
Sleeping pad: https://amzn.to/2VbWKUf
Sleeping bag
Insect repellant
CLOTHING
Workout shoes or boots
Extra socks
Boot bands
Boonie hat or wool cap

	Gloves
	TOOLS
	Emergency Radio: https://amzn.to/2GCTMEJ
	Hand crank Flashlight: https://amzn.to/2Vg1bgK
	Battery powered headlamp: https://amzn.to/2RdecZk
	Signal Mirror: https://amzn.to/2BGKOAy
	VS-17 signal panel: https://amzn.to/2Sqqzyz
	Folding Saw: https://amzn.to/2LwcHQF
	Fishing Kit: https://amzn.to/2BC36TK
	Snares: https://amzn.to/2Lwd6Tb
	Electrical tape
	Candles (per Area Study) useful for glazing snow caves
	Survival axe (per Area Study) also is a weapon: https://amzn.to/2BDuAby
	Machete (per Area Study): https://amzn.to/2CxTgE4
	Snow shovel (per Area Study): https://amzn.to/2RkYNpA
	Pocket chainsaw (per Area Study): https://amzn.to/2BI7YqC

MISC ITEMS	
	Compass: https://amzn.to/2GAOycI
	Assorted zip ties along with Handcuff zip ties: https://amzn.to/2Rdar61
	Map of Area
	Waterproof map case
	Pen, paper, pencil
	Optics (binoculars or telescope—as per Area study)
	CASH
	Apps downloaded from Appendix B
	Toilet paper
	Toothbrush and paste
	Razor and blades
	Camping soap
	Camping towel
	Feminine hygiene products as needed

Task Thirty-Nine. Moderate Hide Site Cache

	Emergency ration bars
	Emergency radio
	Snares
	Shelter (poncho, 550 cord)
	First Aid kit

Appendix B: Useful APPs

Locator Apps

Road ID Here is their home page with links to both Apple and Android along with information on how the app works. https://www.roadid.com/pages/road-id-app	
Life 360 Android: https://play.google.com/store/apps/details?id=com.life360 .android.safetymapd Apple: https://itunes.apple.com/us/app/life360-family-tracker/id384830320?mt=8	
Sygic Family locatorAndroid: https://play.google.com/store/apps/details?id=com.sygic.f amilywhere.android&hl=cs&referrer=utm_source%3Dsyg ic-com%26utm_medium%3Dheader- features%26utm_campaign%3Dfamily-locator Apple: https://itunes.apple.com/sk/app/family-locator-gps-tracker/id588364107?mt=8	

Trusted Contacts: Android: https://play.google.com/store/apps/details?id=com.google. android.apps.emergencyassist&utm_source=google&utm _medium=web&utm_campaign=homepage Apple: https://itunes.apple.com/app/trusted-contacts/id1225684042	

First Aid Apps

	Red Cross First Aid App (Apple): https://itunes.apple.com/us/app/first-aid-by-american-red/id529160691?mt=8 **(Android):** https://play.google.com/store/apps/det ails?id=com.cube.arc.fa&hl=en	
	iTriage App (Apple): https://itunes.apple.com/us/app/itriage -symptom-checker/id304696939 **(Android):** https://play.google.com/store/apps/det ails?id=com.healthagen.iTriage	
	CPR and choking app: (Apple): https://itunes.apple.com/app/cpr-choking/id314907949 **CPR and Choking (Android):** https://play.google.com/store/apps/det ails?id=org.learncpr.videoapp	

5-0 Police Scanner APP (Apple)	https://itunes.apple.com/us/app/5-0-radio-police-scanner/id356336433?mt=8
Fire and Police Scanner APP (Android)	https://play.google.com/store/apps/details?id=com.scannerradio&hl=en_US

Red Cross hurricane app (Apple): https://itunes.apple.com/us/app/hurricane-by-american-red/id545689128?mt=8

Red Cross hurricane app (Android): https://play.google.com/store/apps/details?id=com.cube.arc.hfa&hl=en

Earthquake alert (Android): https://play.google.com/store/apps/details?id=com.joshclemm.android.quake&hl=en

Quake Alert (Apple): https://itunes.apple.com/us/app/quakefeed-earthquake-map-alerts/id403037266?mt=8

Weatherbug (Apple): https://itunes.apple.com/app/weathcrbug-forecasts-radar/id281940292

Weatherbug (Android): https://play.google.com/store/apps/details?id=com.aws.android

Disaster   Alert   (Apple):
https://itunes.apple.com/us/app/disaster-alert-pacific-disaster/id381289235

Disaster   Alert   (Android):
https://play.google.com/store/apps/details?id=disasterAlert.PDC

FEMA   (apple):
https://itunes.apple.com/us/app/fema/id474807486

FEMA   (Android):
https://play.google.com/store/apps/details?id=gov.fema.mobile.android

Flashlight   (Apple):
https://itunes.apple.com/us/app/flashlight-o/id381471023

Flashlight   (Android):
https://play.google.com/store/apps/details?id=com.ihandysoft.ledflashlight.mini

Appendix C: Useful Web Sites

National Geographic 1:24,000 maps: http://www.natgeomaps.com/trail-maps/pdf-quads
USGS maps: http://nationalmap.gov/ustopo/
Home facts: http://www.homefacts.com/
Dams: http://nid.usace.army.mil/cm_apex/f?p=838:12
Association of State Dam Safety: http://www.damsafety.org/
FEMA safe room guidelines web site: https://www.fema.gov/residential-safe-rooms
Red Cross on line First Aid Courses: http://www.redcross.org/take-a-class/first-aid/first-aid-training/first-aid-online
National Geographic Maps: http://www.natgeomaps.com/trail-maps/pdf-quads
USGS Maps: http://nationalmap.gov/ustopo/
List of nuclear power plants: http://www.nrc.gov/reactors/operating/map-power-reactors.html
Pacific Northwest Seismic Network: https://www.pnsn.org/earthquakes/recent

ALL Bob Mayer BOOKS

THE GREEN BERETS

Eyes of the Hammer   Dragon Sim-13   Cut Out
Synbat   Eternity Base   Z: The Final Option
Chasing the Ghost   Chasing the Lost
Chasing the Son

THE DUTY, HONOR, COUNTRY

AREA 51

Area 51   Area 51 The Reply   Area 51 The Mission
Area 51 The Sphinx   Area 51 The Grail   Area 51 Excalibur

Area 51 The Truth   Area 51 Nosferatu   Area 51 Legend
Area 51 Redemption   Area 51 Invasion

ATLANTIS
Atlantis   Atlantis Bermuda Triangle   Atlantis Devils Sea
Atlantis Gate   Assault on Atlantis   Battle for Atlantis

THE CELLAR
Bodyguard of Lies   Lost Girls

NIGHSTALKERS
Nightstalkers   Book of Truths   The Rift
Time Patrol
This fourth book in the Nightstalker book is the team becoming the Time Patrol, thus it's labeled book 4 in that series but it's actually book 1 in the Time Patrol series.

TIME PATROL SERIES
Black Tuesday   Ides of March   D-Day
Independence Day
Fifth Floor   Nine-Eleven   Valentines Day
Hallows Eve

THE SHADOW WARRIORS
(these books are all stand-alone and don't need to be read in order)

The Line   The Gate   Omega Missile   Omega
Sanction   Section Eight

THE PRESIDENTIAL SERIES
The Jefferson Allegiance   The Kennedy
Endeavor

THE BURNERS SERIES
Burners   Prime

THE PSYCHIC WARRIOR SERIES
Psychic Warrior   Psychic Warrior: Project
Aura

STAND ALONE BOOKS:
THE ROCK   I, JUDAS THE 5TH
GOSPEL

BUNDLES (Discounted 2 for 1 and 3 for 1):
Check web site, books, fiction and nonfiction.

COLLABORATIONS WITH JENNIFER CRUSIE
Don't Look Down   Agnes and The Hitman
Wild Ride

NON-FICTION:
The Green Beret Preparation & Survival
Guide: A Common Sense, Step-by-Step Handbook
for Every Emergency
Stuff Doesn't Just Happen I: The Gift of Failure

Stuff Doesn't Just Happen II: The Gift of
Failure
The Novel Writers Toolkit
Write It Forward: From Writer to Bestselling
Author
Who Dares Wins: Special Operations Tactics
for Success

Thank you!

Made in the USA
San Bernardino, CA
07 April 2019